ARE YOU READY?

Stop Wishing It Was *Friday.*

DARREN STEEVES
M.SC., CSEP-CEP
& SUE COMEAU
M.A., CSEP-CEP

MORE PRAISE FOR
Are You Ready? Stop Wishing It Was Friday

"An enjoyable and helpful book that reads like a story, not a textbook, allowing the reader to grasp important concepts in a relatable way."
- Mark de Jonge, Olympic medalist and World Champion paddler; professional engineer

"Thanks so much for shining a much needed light on this conversation. Your book resonated with me on so many levels having personally experienced many of Alex's "real and perceived" work and life stressors. Having implemented several of your suggested strategies to build better coping skills and cognitive function I can say there is indeed a light at the end of the tunnel. Life comes at us at hyper-speed every day and your book will help give people perspective that they are not alone in their challenges and perhaps more importantly that there is a way forward, we're not helpless, we can take charge of our total health with the right support systems and values in place and live the kind of life we imagine for ourselves."
- Greg Caines, CEBS, Partner, Morneau Shepell Ltd.

"A motivating and practical reminder that overall wellness is a life long journey comprised of an infinite series of small steps. A terrific, easy to read handbook for overall wellness in a busy world."
- Keith Abriel, CFO, DHX Media

"This is a story about Alex, and about me, you, all of us. It is an engaging reminder that each of us has the choices and the power to be better aligned with our best selves."
- Janice MacInnis, Manager, Organizational Health Human Resources, Dalhousie University

"Health is not a fad diet or 10 minute abs. It is your entire life. It is being the best version of you. Working towards your best self can be challenging, and sometimes you may fall off course. 'Are you Ready?...' can help you understand how small, health-focused choices can have a tremendous impact on your health and keep you focused on what's important to you."
- Jesse Adams MSc, CSCS, Partner, Vendura Wellness

FOREWORD

Blink once. Blink twice. Blink three times, and before you know it your life has passed you by. The time we have on this earth is short. We all know the deal: there's an ending. This is not news.

What may be news for some is that we really do have a say in how our life turns out; it's not all luck.

Whether we know this or not is not as important as what we do in the end. If we get caught up in 'doing life' versus 'living life', there's more risk for feeling trapped.

Without noticing it, many times this happens because of going on automatic pilot that drives our behavior and focus. Job, bills, job, bills, family, job, bills, and the rare moments of time to focus on self.

When we get caught in autopilot doing life, what may not be obvious is why we are where we are is because of earlier decisions we made, such as job or career, people we hang around with, and the lifestyle choices we make.

When a person goes on autopilot it's often done unconsciously, and the strain of doing versus living life often leads to a common set of feelings and thoughts, such as feeling lost, confused and stressed.

The more one focuses on these kinds of feelings and thoughts, the greater the risk of believing we're trapped.

When this happens, it's not uncommon to look for outlets to feel good or to forget why we do what we do to figure out how to cope better, as we struggle to understand our meaning in life.

The fact is, most of us have never taken a course on the life lesson to be happy. If you're wondering how to get more out of life and are not quite sure how, this is not uncommon. Life can be hard and at times even seem unfair. It's best not to judge yourself but accept that you may not be where you want to be, and be open to finding a different way.

Pause. Stop. Look in the mirror and ask yourself if any of the above makes sense and you can relate to it in any way, whether yourself or someone you love.

The good news is there are options and a pathway to making new decisions that can change your course of life.

Taking time to stop and consider what you can do differently to change, improve, tweak, or evolve provides an opportunity for new awareness, accountability and action to change the course of your life.

Whether it's a small or big change doesn't matter; it starts with one decision at a time.

Are You Ready? Stop Wishing It Was Friday provides an opportunity to look through the eyes of a typical human being who is figuring out how to move from doing life versus living it.

Each chapter allows you to experience and ponder Alex's journey and the opportunities and decisions he's exploring so he can move from doing to living his life.

There's no one path. Some may have one or two areas we can tweak to change our day-to-day experiences.

Each of the 45 chapters is short and easy to read. They provide a narrative and opportunity to find an idea or thought that can help you decide to do something different.

After you read the first section of the book, different themes may jump out. Most will find two or three key themes and ideas that relate to them.

The *Are You Ready?...* Guide is a neat way to review the key theme and lesson for each chapter. This can help connect the dots as to what decisions can be made to improve a theme that can influence and shape how a person lives their life.

The authors' goal is to provide the reader with a wide enough swath of topics to ensure there are a few relevant themes.

Being a human being is complex. Many different themes can come into play to influence our perceptions of how well we are living our life. There's no magic bullet nor formula. This book is meant to be a guide to help people make decisions that can have a positive impact on their life. We each have one life to live, and we make our own decisions that define it.

Are You Ready? Stop Wishing It Was Friday provides an easy and safe way to have a conversation with yourself about where you are today, and if you are in fact living life or doing life. Living life with clear intention and a plan will be more fulfilling than feeling like you're not in control.

One of the most important lessons I've learned after 30 years of working with people is that with good information, guidance and support, they can make better decisions. Happiness and fulfillment happen one decision at a time. Making life change is simply deciding to do a few things differently every day until you achieve your desired outcome, and then evaluating what's next and making a new plan. Living life to its fullest takes focus and energy; there's no escaping this fact.

In the end, making decisions without a clearly-defined action plan seldom is enough. This is perhaps why every year millions of New Year's resolutions fail. To get the most out of this book, once you see one or two areas where you can make better decisions, be clear on how you will act.

Happy decision-making!

William A. Howatt, Ph.D., Ed.D.
Chief of Research and Development, Workforce Productivity
Morneau Shepell

CHAPTER 1

When had I started to feel so bad?

As I leaned back in my chair and stretched, I realized that thought had been nagging at me all week.

I sat upright and looked at the half-full soda on my desk, and the remains of a burger and curly fries, from my favorite burger place. I had wolfed them down fast, and now I burped up the aftertaste.

I patted my chest, where my daily dose of heartburn was starting to simmer. I always say that I can't get enough of those fries. Right now, I had had more than enough.

Taking a deep breath, I looked down at my gut. Man, we used to joke about those guys that couldn't see below the belt anymore; I was becoming one of them.

(When was the last time I even attempted to work out? I couldn't remember.)

It was Friday night and I was working late again. I said I'd take on this proposal – I don't know why.

Was I even getting ahead anymore?

One more email to send, and then I'd be outta here. Checking my phone, I had a vague feeling of disappointment.

This phone was my new toy, the latest version with everything.

Used to be, I'd have a cute little text asking when I'd be home. Now, nothing.

I shook my head, getting the cobwebs out, and tried to focus.

Instead, I found myself staring at a few of the framed pictures on my desk: My wedding picture. My son. Me and my business school buddies. All of us grinning back at me, everyone happy. Was I still happy?

It didn't seem like my life anymore.

I looked up at the pasty white ceiling of my office.

Yeah, I thought again, when did I get to this?

CHAPTER 2

Some people believe in destiny. I don't know.

What I do know is that things aren't always what they seem.

Sometimes a small change becomes a big deal. The girl who annoyed the hell out of you in school becomes the love of your life.

And sometimes a guy who pisses you off on first meeting can turn out to be your best friend. Or your savior. Or both…

It was the end of another sixty-hour work week.

Finally out of the office, I drove home in my little Audi TT. This was another 'toy' I bought a couple of years ago. I loved it, but I also felt like I should have a nice car to, you know, project success.

I pulled into our driveway and shut off the ignition.

All I could think about was a nice cold beer. Or a few.

We had just moved into this house last week.

It was a beautiful historical house in a highly sought after neighborhood. The previous owners had modernized it.

I should have been over the moon.

Hopefully my wife and son were watching a movie or something. It wasn't only the little messages that had stopped. They usually all but ignored me when I got home these days.

I sat for an extra few seconds and looked out my window at the dark, inky sky. I used to love this dusky time of night. Now it just seemed black.

I got out of the car and rubbed my neck. It's chronically screwed up now. I used to try to get to a physical therapist when I could, but that's a rarity these days. Now, I usually just suck it up and deal with the pain.

I jingled my keys, to find the new front door key. All seemed quiet. Good. I love my family, but I just needed to decompress. I didn't feel like talking to anyone. Just a few beers and some TV.

"Hey!" came a booming voice.

I jumped and glanced behind me, startled. I fumbled with my keys and they dropped. (I didn't think I was that edgy!)

I hadn't even looked when I got out of the car. Stupid!

I spun around.

The booming voice was bigger than the guy it belonged to. An older man I had seen around the neighborhood. It was hard to tell how old he was, but he looked incredibly fit. I didn't put him over 55, that's for sure.

I looked at him, then straightened up and sucked in my gut, self-consciously.

"Uh, hey," I stuttered out.

The guy stepped forward toward my keys, but I bent down and grabbed them off the ground first. I stepped back.

"Oh jeez, sorry about that," he said, a little quieter this time. "Didn't mean to surprise you like that."

He thrust his hand forward. "I'm Jim," he said, a little too enthusiastically for my state of mind.

I fumbled with my keys again, switching hands, and shook his. "Alex," I offered shortly.

"So you just moved in," he continued brightly.

My only thought: cold beer.

"Yeah."

Okay, social chitchat was going to end here. I don't need to start a relationship with this guy, I thought. How could I get out of this fast?

"In fact, I should get in the house. Crazy work day, and we have a lot of unpacking to do this weekend."

A teenager biked by. "Hey Jim," he called out.

Jim turned and waved. "Hey Ben! Nice game the other day!"

The kid grinned and called back, "Thanks!"

We had only just moved in, but it was obvious this man knew everyone. He turned his attention back to me.

"Yes, Joanie said everything was upside down," Jim replied.

"You met my wife," I half-asked. (Funny, he used her old nickname.)

"Oh yes, my wife Vanessa and I had a grand chat with Joanie and your little guy. David, right?"

"Yeah," I trailed off.

"He's a sweet kiddo," Jim commented.

"Thanks," I said.

"Hopefully you got some of that apple crisp Vanessa made," he added.

(I hadn't. I had grabbed take out most nights because I was so late.)

"Vanessa's a fantastic cook. She used organic apples and no extra sugar."

"That's great," I said. (I couldn't care less.) "Okay Jim, well, nice to meet you but I'd better get in there."

I pointed to the house then glanced back at him.

He hadn't taken his eyes off me. "I'm glad I met you, Alex," he said warmly. "I hope you have a wonderful evening with your family."

(Or that nice cold beer, I thought.)

I turned toward the house, giving a wave. "You too," I replied.

I glanced back as I put my key in the lock. It was nice of the guy to come over and introduce himself. I had an unsettled feeling; I hoped he didn't make this a regular occurrence. I didn't need extra people in my life right now. I was too busy.

I kind of felt bad though, like I had brushed him off. Or something. There was something strangely familiar about him. I couldn't put my finger on it.

I walked into the house and dropped my keys on the table that Joan had put in the foyer. She had put a little pottery bowl there for keys and stuff. It looked nice.

The tulips in the matching vase she had put beside it were dying. I hadn't really noticed how much she had organized everything.

She was working full time too, picking up David from his after school program, and then cooking supper for them. Just another thing to increase my 'guilt-meter'.

I glanced back out the window beside the front door, as I sat down on a bench to take off my shoes.

Mr. Perky – Jim I think his name was – was sitting on his veranda with some lady. Must be his wife. They were just talking and laughing. I watched them longer than you should watch your neighbors.

I sighed.

This was a year ago, but I can still remember sighing. I was so damn tired.

I could hear the TV on in the basement. I was still getting used to the layout of this place. We had stretched things a little to buy this house – a little bigger, a little nicer, and, we were paying through the nose for this neighborhood.

One thing I knew how to find right away: the fridge.

I went to our oversized, top of the line fridge and grabbed one of the imported beers I had bought.

Uncapping it, I took a good long, refreshing drink. Then another.

I looked at the label. One of the guys at work recommended this one, from Germany. Pretty good.

I should get down there, I thought.

I plodded down the stairs to our basement family room with my drink. The room was huge, but Joan had made it seem cozy. I observed that as if I was a visitor here.

We had a guest room (which I might end up in if I wasn't careful), a wet bar, and a bathroom on this level also.

Joan and David were watching a movie. David was five years old, and such a sweet kid. He couldn't care less if I was around though. He and Joan were a little team, and I was on the bench.

"Hey," I said, trying to sound upbeat.

Nothing.

Joan gave me a half-hearted wave and smile.

"Say hi to Daddy, David," Joan reprimanded.

"Hi," he said sullenly.

"It's the end of the movie," Joan whispered to me.

I went over and sat on the arm of the couch Joan and David were stretched out on. Then I moved over to a chair.

I took another slug of beer and pretended to be interested in the movie. But the truth was, my mind was wandering all over the place – mainly still at work.

Two thoughts kept nagging at me. The first was just how bad I felt. And the second was another reason I didn't have time for that guy, Jim: I think I was jealous.

He had something that I wanted. I just didn't know it yet.

CHAPTER 3

The movie David and Joan were watching was one of those funny Pixar animated movies that kids love, but adults can watch too.

They both laughed at a silly part. I looked at them. David was snuggled into Joan, twirling her hair. I couldn't believe he was already five years old.

Looking at them now, you could see how much he looks like Joan. He's solid like me (well, the way I used to be), but he has Joan's dark wavy hair, and those chocolate brown eyes. He's going to have the girls chasing him, no doubt about it.

Looking at him then, I realized he was growing up way too fast, and I was on the outskirts.

He wasn't a mama's boy, but he and Joan just clicked. He was usually just as happy – or happier - to hang out with her. I was usually working so much, that I just accepted that. But when I stopped to think about how much they did together (even with her working) and how much fun they had, I was wistful.

I missed them. Even when I was with them.

But my job is to provide, and my career is important to me. I've given a lot to get to where I am and where I want to go. I can't always be 'fun dad' and 'attentive husband'.

"You okay Dad?" David was looking at me.

I snapped out of it.

"Yeah buddy," I started. "Just…" I smiled at him.

He smiled back at me, this sincere, sweet expression that made me melt.

It was like he felt bad for me, or was waiting for me to finish something. I couldn't even finish my sentence. He turned back to the movie.

I got up and grabbed another beer, even though I didn't really feel like it. Habit I guess.

I always said that working hard was worth it, if you could afford to buy premium stuff. Problem was, it just didn't taste as good these days.

I plunked myself back in my seat.

In that moment, I realized how low I felt.

The funny thing was, I kept telling myself how lucky I was: beautiful house in a good neighborhood, sweet, healthy kid, beautiful wife, steady job.

But the words didn't sink in.

It was like I was on a treadmill, and I couldn't get off. Or at least I didn't know how to get off.

I felt like shit. I wasn't connecting with my family. I had lost touch with my good friends. I was eating like crap and drinking too much. I hadn't gone to the gym in ages. I was stressed.

Was this it?

I knew I was feeling sorry for myself, but I didn't think I could feel much worse than I did right now.

The movie ended. David and Joan both stretched.

"Okay sweetie pie, time for bed" she said.

"Carry me," he begged.

"What? You're such a big boy," she laughed, as she started to gather up his tired little body.

"Can I carry you up, buddy?" I asked.

David hesitated. "Uh," he started.

Joan looked at me. I could see pity in her eyes.

"I'll bet Dad will piggy back you," she said, giving him a smooch.

"Or I'll carry you like a lumberjack," I laughed, popping David over my shoulder.

He was laughing too. When we all got upstairs, I was pretty winded from two flights of stairs.

I pulled him off my shoulder and gave him a bear snuggle, then I let him bounce down onto his bed. Man, I thought, I love this kid.

I had to get it together.

I would take David to the park tomorrow. Maybe take them both out for lunch. We could do a little work in the yard, set up a swing for David in the backyard. Maybe Joan and I would get a movie tomorrow night.

Joan looked at me. "Your mother called," she informed me. "They're coming to visit tomorrow."

I was wrong: I could feel worse.

CHAPTER 4

I grew up in a small town, a couple of hours away from here.

It was the classic old-fashioned upbringing: Dad worked as a supervisor in the local factory. He was really well-respected, and just a stoic guy.

Mom had been a nurse, but she quit once I was born. She stayed at home with my little sister, my little brother, and me. They're two and four years younger than me, respectively.

Being the oldest, I was expected to set the example, get good grades, the whole deal. I always felt the pressure to do well. Mom was always going on about how hard Dad worked to help us out for university.

Mom said she just wanted us to get a good education and 'make something of ourselves'. What she really wanted was a doctor in the family, or a lawyer or engineer.

Meanwhile, Dad was volunteering on the weekends, hauling us around to too many sports (which I hated), and working on house projects all the time.

Dad's always been a no emotion kind of guy. He was a great provider, financially. I don't remember ever hugging my dad.

Mom was always the master of the guilt trip. (She still is.) Maybe that's why news of their visit gave me heartburn.

Or maybe I was having a heart attack.

I fleetingly thought, maybe if I'm in the hospital, they won't come.

But here I was, sitting out on our front doorstep with David, awaiting their arrival.

We have a wide, covered porch, which Joan had bought rocking chairs for, but we were both hunched over on the step.

David looked bored, and I wasn't even sure what to talk to him about.

It was 9:55, and so they would be here in exactly five minutes. Exactly. Dad has always been meticulously on time.

Joan was in the house, cleaning like crazy. She'd heard my mother's well-meaning but condescending comments before.

Last night, as David was brushing his teeth, I asked her why they were coming.

"Your mother needs to do some shopping," she'd replied, her voice edgy.

"Are they staying overnight?" I had asked.

"Yes," she tried to say calmly.

That meant that Joan had busted her butt to organize the guest room, and clean it. Just another thing that she didn't want to deal with yet.

"I'm sorry, but…" I trailed off.

She had waved me away. "They're your parents, Alex. Don't be sorry." But she didn't look at me.

"I just don't understand why they didn't stay at Emily's house," I went on.

"Mommy! I need toilet paper," David had called out.

Joan shook her head. She was trying not to say anything, but I knew she was pissed off, thinking the same thing.

"Just a sec," she'd called back to David. "I'll get some."

Then, to me, "I don't know."

And off she went.

My sister, Emily, lives twenty minutes away, and has always been my parents' pride and joy. She's a dermatologist, has a ten year old daughter and eight year old twins, and is married to Glen, a vascular surgeon. So Mom got her doctor.

I might as well tell you now, my little brother, Richard, is an environmental engineer. So, yeah, another notch in my mother's apron. He travels all over the world, one of the guys who saves the day when there's a big environmental disaster. He's racked up so many air miles, he flew my parents to Europe last year.

My folks still can't figure out what I do with my business degree. Being a consultant isn't saving the world.

9:58.

They would be driving up the street in a minute.

I saw Jim, that guy I met last night, coming out of his house with a bike helmet and a backpack on. He saw me and waved. I waved back.

"Hi Jim!" David was waving wildly at him.

"Hey David," he called back. He gave him a big wave. "What're you up to today?" He grabbed a bike from the side of his house but waited for an answer.

"Nothing," David yelled back.

I looked at David, then at Jim. "My parents are coming," I called out.

"Fantastic," Jim said, hopping on his bike.

Then to David he said, "You remind me after your visit, and I'll show you and your folks the bike trails. Okay David?"

"Awesome!"

With a wave, he cycled off down the street.

"Jim's really cool," David told me.

"Yeah," I agreed.

Then he got quiet again.

Last night, bringing David upstairs and tucking him in, I thought we could have a nice, relaxing weekend. I had been thinking of getting out our bikes, maybe barbequing.

Man, it seemed like every time I felt like I was coming out of the proverbial hole, and starting to feel like I could get ahead, something else happened.

10:00.

Right on cue, Dad's Ford sedan drove up the street.

I turned to David. "Could you tell Mom that Gramma and Grampa are here?"

He got up and went in.

Trying to force a smile, I had to tell myself to unclench my jaw.

My weekend, like my life, was out of my control.

CHAPTER 5

It should be a nice thing to have your parents visit. But as I saw my mother eye the house as they pulled to a stop in front of it, I could see judgment already. Nothing was ever good enough.

I knew that drove Joan crazy too.

Plus, I had just effectively lost my weekend. Any thoughts of relaxing were out the window.

David came back out and put his hand up in a little wave. We both stood up as Mom and Dad got out of the car.

I noticed Dad was a little heavier, moving a little slower. Whenever we were home, sitting around the TV, having a few beers, he'd pat his stomach and say, "I've earned this."

"How's my boy?" That was Mom talking to David, as she extracted herself from the big sedan.

We stepped off the porch and went to greet them.

"Hi Gramma," David said, in that sweet voice of his, as my mother hugged him.

"Oh my, David, look how big you are," Mom exclaimed.

"Yeah, I'm going to be in school soon," he informed her proudly.

He was so cute, and growing up way too fast. I wanted to just pick him up and take him somewhere and hang out for the whole weekend, just with him. I instantly felt guilty for not being able to.

My Dad stepped around and shook his little hand, then patted him on the back.

"There's my guy," Dad said, tousling his hair.

"Hi Grampa," he followed.

Mom hugged me and looked at the house again. "It's nice," she said. "Are you all settled in?"

"Yeah, Joan's done an amazing job," I started, as Dad shook my hand.

"We had a little trouble finding this place," Dad informed me. He turned toward the house too, then scanned the street. "Good neighborhood?"

I nodded. Joan came out on the doorstep and down the walkway.

"Hi Linda, hi Tim," she said warmly. "Welcome!"

Joan could turn it on, the charm I mean, which I appreciated right now.

Mom hugged her and more 'how are you's were passed back and forth. Dad did what passed for his hug: a couple of pats on the back.

"Well come on in and see our new place," Joan invited. "Here guys, let's help Gramma and Grampa with their bags."

Dad popped the trunk and got out one small overnight bag, and a small suitcase for my mother. She also had her big purse and another tote. There were a couple of shopping bags too. Just enough to clutter up our newly organized house once we got it in.

"I don't want to leave those shopping bags in the trunk," she told my father.

"It's a pretty safe neighborhood, Mom," I offered.

"Still," she sniffed.

So we all went in, carrying her stuff.

"Here Gramma," David said, grabbing her purse and slinging it over his shoulder. It looked like a duffel bag on him.

He was such a little gentleman. Sadly, Joan had probably taught him that. I wasn't around enough to.

We got in the house, and plunked down my parents' stuff.

"David, why don't you help Daddy show Gramma and Grampa our new house," Joan said, picking him up.

"Okay, want to see my room?"

David led them up the wide oak staircase to the second floor. I looked at Joan.

"I'll make lunch," she said, trying to sound positive. Then she turned away from me.

Back when we were first married, we used to go for a walk in the park on Saturday mornings, then pop into one of the local bakeries for fresh rolls, and grab the weekend papers. Then we'd put on a pot of coffee and spend the rest of the morning lazing around. Even when David was little, we'd bring him with us in the stroller.

Truth was, we really needed a weekend to relax and settle in.

My folks came downstairs with David.

"It's nice," Mom said. "Just three bedrooms?"

"That's all we need," I said, trying to keep my voice light. "Plus, they're pretty big, and we have an attic office."

"We have another guest room downstairs, Linda," Joan told her patiently. "I thought you and Tim would be comfortable there."

"I'm just saying, when Emily picked out her house, she got five bedrooms, in case they had more kids," Mom started. "Then along came the twins."

She said that as if this stuff was magic. Joan and I were lucky to have David.

Mom looked at David. "Wouldn't you like to have a brother or sister?"

Oh. My. God.

We were in the kitchen now, so Joan got to hear.

"I want a puppy," David replied.

Beautiful.

Dad stepped in. "Linda, I don't think now is the time."

I mouthed 'thank you' to Dad.

"Come and see our back yard," David said excitedly, as he led them toward the French doors.

I followed too. I glanced at Joan on the way by. I think she was gritting her teeth. Even a couple of years ago, I would have been able to joke around with her about the craziness of our parents. But now I just walked by her and whispered, "sorry."

We went out on the back deck, then a couple of steps into the patio and yard. We stood under the big maple tree. This was one of my favorite things about the yard.

"I hope this doesn't make your yard too shady," Mom said. "Emily got landscape designers in."

"Well Mom, Emily and Glen are pulling in well over a million and a half dollars a year," I shot back.

"I'm just saying, you don't want a damp backyard," Mom said defensively.

"Dad's going to make me a swing," David bragged.

"That's lovely sweetheart," Mom half-said to David.

Then to me, as if I was a five year old, "It's very nice."

"Mom, we're not even settled in yet," I commented.

"I'm just trying to be helpful," Mom said indignantly.

"Linda, cut the boy some slack," he half-joked.

"Dad's not a boy," David laughed.

"You're our good boy, aren't you David," Dad said as he took his hand.

I took a deep breath and looked up at the sky. Why couldn't they have picked a different weekend to visit?

"Now, let's take a look at the rest of your house," he boomed. "You gonna offer your old man a beer?"

"Tim, it's not even noontime," Mom scolded.

"It's noon somewhere," Dad laughed. "Am I right, Alex?"

He started heading back toward the house just as Joan came out. "Lunch is ready," she said, trying to sound happy about it.

"Great. Then I've got to take your mother to the mall," Dad informed me, rolling his eyes. "Why don't you and David come?"

"Actually, Alex, there's a neighborhood barbeque tomorrow afternoon. We need a few things," Joan said. "If you're going, I'll make a list."

"Neighborhood barbeque," I repeated, questioningly.

"Yes, someone just came by when you were in the yard, to make sure we knew," Joan told me. "It's potluck. I'd really like to go, and it will be good for David to meet some of the neighborhood kids."

"Yay!" Okay, so obviously David wanted to go too.

I've always been a social guy, but right now, the thought of standing around someone's yard, meeting a ton of new people, then having to remember who everyone was, just made me feel tired and, frankly, a little anxious!

My weekend was effectively out of my control.

CHAPTER 6

After lunch, I found myself heading to my version of Hell: the mall.

Dad drove while Mom babbled on in the front seat. David and I sat in the back seat. Somehow - even though I'm thirty-five, with a wife, kid, house, and career – I felt like I was twelve years old again.

By the time we started circling the parking lot, my blood pressure was sky high, I'm sure. The folks had to have the closest parking space they could get.

I'll skip the details, but here are the highlights of the mall:

I picked up the nine things on Joan's list.

I listened to Dad give me (the business management consultant) advice on how to invest my tax savings - courtesy of Emily's husband (the surgeon).

No irony there.

I ate an ice cream sundae, then finished off David's when Dad decided we should go to the food court.

I wasn't even hungry, but Dad was so insistent, and David was so excited to get a treat. Besides, I tend to eat when I'm stressed, and this was as good a time as any!

I sat on a bench with Dad and David, waiting (seemingly forever) for Mom to finish shopping.

Oh yeah, and I got jostled a couple of times by groups of teenagers, who obviously had nothing better to do than troll the mall. That stuff would have never bugged me before. I don't know why it did now.

By the time we came out and walked back to the car, David was tired and grumpy. And frankly, so was I. Plus I felt like crap after eating that sundae that I hadn't been hungry for.

It was a beautiful, sunny afternoon, and I had spent it at the mall.

"I need a beer," Dad stated.

So did I.

When we pulled in the driveway, I could see that neighbor, Jim, doing some gardening on his front lawn. We got out and started unloading Mom's bags and my stuff. David ran inside.

"Oh my good lord," Dad said, running his hand along the side of the car.

"What's wrong, Dad?" I asked.

"Look at this," Dad started. "How did I miss this?"

It was a scratch on the lower part of the driver's side door.

"Look at that gouge in the paint," Dad said, showing me. "Someone must have done that at the mall."

"It doesn't look too bad," I started.

"The whole door will have to be painted," Dad went on.

Mom had put her hand up to her mouth, as if this all was some sort of catastrophe.

Jim must have looked over and noticed, because he was heading across the street towards us.

"Is everything okay?" Jim asked as he got to us.

"Someone gouged my car," Dad informed him. "I think it's dented a little too. That's going to cost a few hundred to repair."

Jim took a look. "Oh yes, I see it," he said, nodding. "Thank goodness it's not more serious."

Dad looked at him blankly.

"You know, it's money, and a hassle, but," he trailed off.

Dad just looked at his car.

"Do you have a good body shop guy?" Jim asked.

Dad shook his head. "Yeah, but he charges an arm and a leg."

"I can give you a name of a friend here who's very reasonable," Jim followed. "He's a mechanic, but he loves painting and detailing cars on the side. He's quite good."

"Jim," I broke in. "These are my parents, Linda and Tim. They're just visiting for tonight."

They shook hands. "It's good to meet you," Jim said. Dad echoed the sentiment, but was distracted by his car.

"So this seems like a nice neighborhood?" Mom asked.

"Oh yes," Jim assured her. "Alex, Joanie and David will be very happy here. We've got a nice park, it's walking distance to everything, and the people here are wonderful."

Jim turned to me. "You're all coming to the barbeque tomorrow? Your folks are welcome too."

"That sounds lovely," my mother said to Jim. Then she turned to me. "But we promised Emily we would stop by on the way home. She's having a catered dinner for us."

"Well, it was nice to meet you," Jim said sincerely. "Next time."

Dad stood up again. "Good to meet you, Jim. Sorry it's under these circumstances."

Jim looked confused for a second, then Dad motioned to the scratch on the door.

"Yes, good to meet you. Luckily that's fixable," Jim said with a wave. "Let me know if you want that name."

And he was off across the street.

I wanted to follow him.

Instead, I followed Mom and Dad into the house, Dad grumbling about the mall and the hassle of getting the paint job fixed.

That night, I did the usual: I ate too much, I drank more than I wanted, I sat and watched the game on TV with Dad for way too long, and then I went to bed and slept like crap, as usual.

My acid reflux was driving me crazy, probably due to the food and alcohol, or maybe it was the anxiety. On the roulette wheel of feeling bad these days, who knew!

Usually, when I attempted to have a decent sleep, work stress was the culprit that kept me awake. I couldn't turn my brain off.

This week, another thought kept sneaking in:

Is this what my life is all about?

CHAPTER 7

The next morning, we had a big breakfast with Mom and Dad. Every meal was a food fest with my family.

Then, thankfully, they were on their way.

I wasn't sure how much more small-town gossip and bragging about Emily Joan could take.

After we waved my parents off, Joan announced she and David were going to go to her friend's place for a 'playdate'. The kids play and the mothers drink coffee and chat, I guess. Probably complain about their husbands. I think it was a buddy of David's from preschool.

Joan and I weren't exactly sharing intricate details of our days with each other these days, so I wasn't sure.

Anyway, they high-tailed it out, and I had a couple of hours to clean and organize the garage. The lawn needed a mow too. Plus I had about five other major things on the list that I hadn't gotten to. There's always a list.

The couple of hours flew by, and when Joan and David got back, it was almost time to go to the barbeque.

I cleaned up and grabbed a bottle of wine. I poured myself a stiff drink while Joan finished getting ready. I felt I needed it to get through this event. I looked down at the empty glass and it struck me: What am I doing??

Joan came down the stairs and grabbed the salad she had made. It looked delicious. I couldn't remember the last time she had made a salad. Sure, she usually got veggies and dip for David, for school lunches. But we didn't exactly eat like health gurus these days.

Anyway, David was bouncing around, loving life.

At five, a lot of kids are pretty shy, but not David. He's always been a really outgoing kid. I used to joke that he got it from me.

"Where are we going?" I asked as we all walked up the street together.

"It's three houses up, the Johnsons," Joan said, not looking at me. I glanced over at her. I knew she didn't feel great these days. Work was stressing her out. She had put on a few pounds (her words not mine), and she never smiled anymore. Well, not at me anyway.

We got to the house, and there was a sign on the back gate, telling everyone to 'Come on in!'

We walked through, into a nice grassy yard, with a big tree similar to ours. They had chairs and assorted lawn furniture dispersed around the lawn and the patio. A few kids were playing with soccer balls in a corner of the yard.

Within about thirty seconds, we were enveloped by a lot of friendly faces.

A woman stepped forward. "Joanie! David! So glad you made it! And you must be Alex," she said warmly. She hugged them, and then extended her hand to shake mine.

She was super tall. I'm six feet. She had to be six two.

"Hi Kim," David said excitedly, and then he ran over to join some other kids.

"Alex, this is Kim Johnson," Joan said happily.

"It's a pleasure to meet you," I smiled. Then an even taller guy came over and put his arm around Kim.

These two had to be basketball players.

"Hey guys, welcome," he said smoothly. "I'm Ty, Kim's better half." He braced for the inevitable elbow from her, and started laughing. "Joanie and Alex, right?"

I nodded and we shook hands. He took the salad off Joan's hands for her. "Looks great," he said.

"I've got to ask," I started.

"Yeah, we both played varsity basketball at Boston College," he answered.

"That's how we met," she added.

We laughed. "Obviously you get that question a lot," Joan said, grinning.

Kim and Ty introduced us to a few others right away. "We don't want to overwhelm you," Kim laughed.

Then they led us further into the yard and showed us where the drinks were. The yard was beautiful, as if they spent a lot of time using it.

Everyone was super friendly. It looked like a really great bunch of neighbors. They also looked, honestly, pretty fit and healthy. I looked down at myself and felt a pang of anxiety. I could use another drink right now.

A little while later, I saw Jim under one of the trees, chatting with a young guy. He noticed me, ended his conversation, and came over.

"Hey Alex," he smiled. "Are you having fun?"

"Yeah," I said simply, nodding. I actually was having fun.

"It's a great group of people on this street," he agreed. Changing the subject, he asked, "Did your folks get off okay?"

"Yes they did," I said. "I'm sorry about my dad. He's a really good guy. He just hates it when he has to deal with pain in the ass stuff with his car. He doesn't handle stress well."

"No worries," Jim bounced back. "Most people don't. I never used to."

"You seem pretty relaxed," I said, skeptically.

"Ask my wife Vanessa sometime," he laughed. "But I learned something big: You're never going to get rid of stress. Stress is always there. It's how you deal with it that changes everything."

He took out a card. "That's the name of the friend who does painting and body work."

"Thanks," I started.

I felt like a light bulb had just turned on over my head. Jim made a good point. I wanted to talk to him some more. The annoyingly upbeat attitude was growing on me.

"And my number is on there too," he added. "If you have any questions."

(It was like he read my mind!)

"So Jim," I asked. "I didn't even ask. What do you do?"

He laughed. "Oh boy, that's a complicated question these days. I've probably got my hand in a few too many things!"

Then he said, "What are you passionate about?"

"Uh," I stuttered.

That was kind of a weird question. And frankly, I didn't know the answer. "Nothing really."

"Hey Jim!" It was a woman, standing by the long table. "This fruit salad is amazing!"

"You've got to have it with the orange sauce," he called back. "That makes it unbelievable!"

He patted my shoulder. "I'm glad you're here." And he was off toward the table, and presumably, the sauce.

Ty sidled up beside me. "Isn't Jim amazing," he said.

"He is," I said.

"So down to earth," Ty commented.

"Yeah, I guess," I agreed.

Kim called to him, and Ty was off to grab more drinks for everyone, leaving me wondering what the deal was with this guy, Jim.

CHAPTER 8

On the way home, later that afternoon, Joan looked really happy. She was glowing, and she looked great.

I should have told her, but David wanted a shoulder ride, and Joan and I hadn't really talked a lot lately. It seemed weird to say, "you look beautiful," when we hadn't had a good conversation in weeks.

When we got home, I played a game with David. David had some mac and cheese for supper, and Joan and I each sipped a beer while sitting with him and picking at some bread. I was pretty full still.

David gave us some pretty detailed profiles of the neighborhood kids.

"Yeah, so that guy, Jack," he informed us, "he's got two hamsters, Butch and Rocko, but then they had baby hamsters, so now Rocco is Rockella."

"You know those twins, Patrick and Will? They don't even own a TV!"

And on and on…

"And there's a girl called Madison who can do a backflip!" Then, as an afterthought, "She has two moms."

"Oh yeah, I think I met them," I said.

"Oh yeah, me too," Joan added. "Lila and Patty?"

"Yeah, they're cool," David confirmed.

David had become this observant, smart kid, who was so engaging.

After supper I went up with David for his bath, while Joan got lunches ready for the next day.

Of course, he wanted Joan to read to him, so I went back downstairs and grabbed a drink. Just one rum and Coke, to take the edge off.

As usual, stress was already creeping in ahead of Monday. These nice relaxing days never lasted long.

I parked myself in front of the TV and turned on the football game.

A little while later, I woke up in my chair. I looked at my watch. Almost one a.m. All the lights were out.

Joan was probably pissed. She hated it when I fell asleep in front of the TV.

The next morning, I was at work, staring bleary-eyed at my computer. It was seven a.m.

I thought about yesterday afternoon. The neighborhood potluck had been unexpectedly pleasant. David had loved it, and Joan was in a better mood than she'd been for weeks. So was I.

But then the reality of Monday morning hit, and here I was.

I finished replying to the bunch of emails that had come in from clients over the weekend, then sat back in my chair.

I reached for the uneaten half of the breakfast sandwich I had picked up as I swung through the drive-thru. It was cold now. Probably my coffee was too.

I shook my head and re-focused.

Yesterday was fun, but these people must not have demanding jobs or money issues, or anything. This sounds childish, but, sitting at my desk, it kind of bugged me that they were so relaxed and positive. It was like something out of a heartwarming television sitcom.

And I felt like I was just scraping by, in all areas.

What are you passionate about, Jim had said.

Yeah right.

That question had made me feel excited and depressed, all at once. That sounds funny, but it did.

That was partly because I remember being passionate about things. Back when I was in business school, I was the king of ideas. I played a lot of sports. I was involved.

I could imagine the possibilities.

And partly because I couldn't remember the last time I felt excited about something, without it scaring the hell out of me: David. Our new house.

Vacations were even stressful. We usually did an all-inclusive beach trip. It always took me about three days to relax, then by the last couple of days I was stressed, thinking about work again. Then I would think about how much money we had spent for a week.

That evening after work, I had a dinner with clients. I usually don't mind work dinners, but the rich food and booze does a number on me. I never sleep well afterward. After the last dinner, I had to pile about three pillows under my head, because the heartburn was so bad.

I wished I could have been home with Joan and David, picking at mac and cheese and bread, and hearing David's observations about his day and the people in it. Talking to Joan. Just being there.

When I got to the house, I knew David and Joan would be asleep. As I put my key in the door, I turned to look across the street. There were a couple of soft lights on at Jim's house. It looked warm and cozy.

I walked in, and saw the card Jim had given me, with the car guy's number. I picked it up and turned it over.

Jim's number was there, as he said, in case I needed anything.

More and more lately, I was realizing that I did. I needed something.

CHAPTER 9

A couple of weeks passed by, seemingly in a flash.

As a business consultant, there's always a pull to work more; and to keep your clients, as well as the people working under you, happy.

You want to have that edge.

And, although I felt pretty inept in the rest of my life these days, work was going well. My clients were happy, and I was rising to the top at work. We were all dragged out and felt like death warmed over, but we were kicking ass.

Our office is in the heart of downtown, with no lack of pubs and restaurants.

So, with the client dinners and other social stuff, my work buddies and I went out for lunch a few times a week, or for a quick drink after work, just to wind down.

It was good to catch up with these guys, hear who was doing what, etc. You felt like you were on top of the business gossip. Plus, we always talked about what was going on in the markets, etc.

Today was one of those days. It was a Monday, and I was sitting out on one of the restaurant patios, with two of my closest co-workers, Will and Bryan.

Bryan is about five years older than me, divorced, with two kids. He's a workhorse, consistently scoring amazing year-ends.

Will graduated from business school two years behind me, and is super savvy. He's just one of those guys who makes excellent decisions when it really counts. Will got married a few years ago. He and his wife, Ashley, are really fun to hang out with. (I tried to think of the last time we did something with them.)

We were just finishing up some nachos and a beer.

"How's the new house," Bryan boomed to me, more a statement than a question.

"It's great," I said, meaning it. "We're finally feeling settled in."

"Are you living near the park?" Will asked.

"Yeah," I answered, feeling pretty upbeat. "It's a really cool neighborhood. Everyone has been awesome. Joan and David know pretty much everybody now."

"And is your little guy in school this year?" Will asked.

"Starting in 'big school' in September," I said, shaking my head at how quickly he got to five years old.

"They're so sweet at that age," Bryan smiled. "They don't want too much from you. My kids are always asking for money, clothes, the latest phone. Once they hit twelve, they're all about 'keeping up with the Joneses'."

"Really?" I asked. I knew Bryan had a pretty standard custody agreement with his wife. He worked more than me, so I couldn't imagine that left a lot of time with his kids.

"Ah, they're good kids," he said, and trailed off.

We were all sitting back now. We had ordered large nachos, and I had definitely eaten my share.

We all checked our phones, for about the tenth time.

The waitress came by and we all ordered coffees.

"How are things with you and Ashley?" I asked. Will's wife was starting to get antsy in the family department.

"Well, let me tell you, trying to get pregnant is the biggest libido crusher ever. I never thought I'd say this, but sex is like a job now," he told us grimly.

"Oh, poor baby," Bryan quipped.

We all laughed, Will despite himself.

"It'll happen," Bryan counseled. "Just, for God's sake, have some fun! In a couple of years, she won't want to look at you."

(That was a little harsh.)

He laughed again. Will just smiled and shrugged.

Bryan got up to go to the bathroom, giving Will a hearty pat on the shoulder on the way by.

"Did you get the invitation for the alumni get together?" Will asked.

I checked my email.

"Oh yeah, there it is," I nodded.

"I think I'm going to go," Will said. "How about you?"

"Yeah, I'll see," I said tentatively.

Our business school has an awesome alumni and mentoring program.

"I should probably be showing my face at home more as it is," I added.

"I miss those days," Will commented.

"I hear you," I agreed.

Bryan came back and plunked down like a bear. Our coffees arrived.

"So, what's new with the ladies' man?" I joshed.

"I have met someone new," Bryan informed us. "She works out at my gym."

"I thought you were dating Lynn," Will asked.

"I was, but she wanted a ring on her finger," Bryan answered. "I don't need two ex-wives!"

We laughed. I looked at my watch.

"Alright boys," Bryan announced. "We should get back to the trenches."

We agreed. I turned to signal the waitress.

"I got it," Bryan informed us. "One of you get the next one." He changed his voice to high-pitched. "And I want to go to an expensive place next time!"

We laughed and got up.

I was stiff from sitting. I stretched.

Bryan patted me on my gut. "Okay, that's enough working out for today," he chortled. Then to Will, "Alex will make us look bad."

CHAPTER 10

We started walking, slowly, off the pub patio.

"Back to the grind," I said.

And it did feel like a grind these days.

I saw Jim, my neighbor, walking by on the other side of the street.

"I'll see you back at the office, guys," I informed Bryan and Will, waving.

"No window shopping," Bryan joked, and they headed back.

"Jim," I called out, across the street.

Jim was walking at a pretty good clip. He turned and looked.

I waved. "Hey," I called out again.

He waved back. "Hey Alex," he called, in his usual positive tone. He hesitated, the way people do when they're not sure whether you want them to stop and chat, or just keep going.

I waved to him again and started crossing the street. He waited.

I trotted over to Jim.

"I wanted to say thanks for that info," I told him. "The body shop guy."

"Oh sure, my pleasure," he smiled.

I rubbed my chest. I hoped I had some more antacid in my desk drawer.

"You okay, Alex?" he asked.

"Oh, yeah," I said sheepishly. "Nachos for lunch, with jalapenos. That stuff never agrees with me."

"Yes, good going down, but," he trailed off, good-naturedly.

I nodded. "So, what are you doing in these parts?" I asked. "Do you work downtown?"

He laughed. "I volunteer at the YMCA, a few streets over."

From my impatient initial impression of Jim, I found myself welcoming chances to chat in the neighborhood. I wasn't the only one, it seemed. It wasn't hard to realize that everyone in our neighborhood loved the guy. (And his wife.)

"I wonder if you'd have time to meet for lunch sometime," I asked. "Maybe this week?"

If he was surprised at the invitation, he didn't show it. "Sure," he said gamely. "You name the day."

"Great," I started.

"But how about a walk and talk," he broke in. "I'll bring lunch."

"Uh," I stuttered. "Geez Jim, I'm happy to buy lunch. Any favorite restaurants downtown here?"

"Let me bring lunch this time. I'd appreciate it," he countered. "My back acts up when I sit too long."

Somehow, I knew this wasn't the reason.

"Okay, but I could bring," I started again.

"You get it next time," he interrupted. "Just text me later on today, and we can meet outside your office. You've still got my number?"

"Yes, absolutely," I said. I knew when to concede.

"Looking forward to it," he said warmly, as he turned to go.

I waved and stood there for an extra moment as he strode off.

CHAPTER 11

That night when I got home, David was already asleep. Shit. I hated to miss saying goodnight.

"Don't wake him up," Joan said shortly, when I walked into the kitchen, on my way to David's room. "He had soccer tonight, and he was exhausted."

I put my hand on my forehead. "Ah shoot, I forgot."

"Yeah," Joan muttered as she wiped the counter.

"Why didn't you text me?"

She turned to me. "Would it have mattered? Your job always trumps everything else these days."

"I'm sorry Joan," I shot back, "but I'm trying to provide for you here."

She cut me off. "That's you, not us."

"What?"

"Nothing."

Joan turned away, toward the sink.

"No, if you have something to say, say it," I said, a little pissed off now.

"If you want to put your career first, that's your deal," Joan told me. "But don't hide behind the 'I have to provide for you' crap. Face it Alex, you're married to your work these days. Not me. And frankly, it's you, and it's David who are losing out. I'm so used to you not being around, I don't care anymore."

You could have knocked me over with a feather. Joan has always hated conflict. For her to say that, she was really mad.

"I'm around," I started.

"You show up when you really need to show up. But I think you checked out a while ago. And I've gotten over missing the old you already."

She walked past me, out of the kitchen.

The old me?

I went to the cupboard and grabbed a nice bottle of scotch I had been saving. Saving for what, I wondered to myself. I grabbed a glass and a few ice cubes.

Then I sat down at the table with my drink, alone.

A little later, I texted Jim, asking if tomorrow was too soon for lunch.

We made a plan to meet at one o'clock.

CHAPTER 12

The next day, I regretted it for a moment.

I was running behind after back-to-back meetings with clients.

At 12:30, I considered texting Jim to reschedule, but I figured he was on his way. We could make it short.

When I got outside, out of our office air-conditioning, it was a beautiful, sunny day.

Jim was there, on time. He was chatting to an older guy in a suit. He seemed to know a lot of people.

He had a backpack, but looked pretty casual. Did he work from home, I wondered? Or had he taken early retirement?

I blinked in the bright sunlight. He looked my way.

I waved, walking toward him. He acknowledged me, and patted the other man on the shoulder. They shook hands. Then he waved and started toward me.

"How are you, Alex?" he asked. "What a day, huh?"

"It's beautiful," I agreed. "Look, I hope I'm not taking you away from anything today."

"Not at all," he smiled. "Let's walk over this way. Do you ever go to the little park over here?" He pointed past me.

"Uh, no," I admitted.

"A new discovery then," he stated, and we started walking.

We chatted about surface stuff on the way over, about the weather, that it was supposed to be a long, hot summer, and within a few minutes, we were at this green space.

"Wow," I exclaimed. "This is nice."

He nodded. "It's such a gem," he agreed. "And it could be used so much more by people downtown."

Jim pointed to a couple of benches and tables.

"I'm starving," he exclaimed. "Want to sit here?"

"Sure. But Jim, I feel bad," I said good-naturedly. "I invited you to lunch, and you brought everything."

"It's my pleasure," he answered brightly.

We sat down and he unloaded his backpack. He took out a couple of sandwiches, a big bottle of water with a couple of cups, and a container with fruit.

"So, how was your morning?" I asked.

He lit up. "It was great," he said. "Vanessa and I rode that bike trail." He snapped his fingers. "I promised David I'd show him the trail. Just let me know when you have time to come on out. Once you've found it the first time, it's easy."

He handed me a sandwich.

"Sure," I replied. "I don't have a good bike, but I could bring David's."

"Do you know how to ride?" he asked, as he poured the water into two cups.

"Oh yeah," I answered, a little defensively. "I just need a new bike."

"Well, if you want to take David out, just borrow mine sometime," he said agreeably.

I unwrapped the sandwich. It looked like some sort of tomato and cheese. "Thanks for these," I started, then took a bite.

Wow.

"Oh man," I said, surprised. "This is amazing!"

He took a bite of his. "It's tomato, pesto, and fresh mozzarella, on focaccia bread," he said proudly. "We made the pesto."

I nodded, mouth momentarily full.

"How was your morning?" he asked, genuinely interested.

"Ugh, the usual grind," I told him. "My first meeting showed up late, and ran late. Then it all went downhill from there."

"So you're a consultant," Jim half-asked, half-stated.

"Yes, how did you know?"

"Joanie told me. So, it sounds like you deal with some of the larger companies?"

"Yes," I answered. "I'm a solutions guy, basically."

I took another bite. "Wow, this is really fantastic, Jim!"

I had a sip of water. It was wonderful! (I know what you're thinking: It's water!)

"This water," I said. "Is it water?"

Jim laughed.

"We infuse water with different fruit," Jim told me. "Which is a fancy way of saying that we chuck some slices of lime, or orange, or berries in it, and put it in the fridge. It really makes it nice, hey?"

I nodded, my mouth full of another bite of sandwich.

This was really pleasant. I felt like my blood pressure had already come down a few notches. Jim was so easygoing.

"Okay, I've got to ask," I finally said. "What do you do?"

Jim laughed.

I jokingly cringed. So many people say that you shouldn't ask someone what they do for a living. That in these days of political correctness, they might feel labeled. Or something.

"I'm sorry," I followed. "It's just that you seem to have it all together."

"No," Jim chuckled again. "No offence taken. I'm actually retired."

"Oh," I nodded. "Early retirement?"

Jim grinned. "A little early. But I'm seventy five."

My jaw could have hit the ground.

"I loved what I did though. So, to answer your question, I was a consultant too," Jim followed. "Just like you."

CHAPTER 13

Once I recovered from the shock that Jim was about fifteen or twenty years older than he looked, we talked some more.

We had the fruit that he had brought, then walked along the path on the perimeter of the park.

"Does Joan know that you were a consultant?" I asked.

"I don't think she asked," Jim answered. "Why?"

"She thinks you and Vanessa are amazing," I said. "It would just be another thing to live up to." I chuckled self-consciously.

"Yeah?" he asked, leading me to keep talking.

"Well, it's just that, you know, the job is stressful, there's always pressure to work more, I'm never quite living up to expectations at home, let alone doing anything for myself anymore," I ranted. "I feel like crap."

I stopped myself and took a deep breath.

"Sorry," I said, smiling at Jim.

"Don't be sorry," he replied. "I was exactly the same way."

"Then you got it together when you retired," I nodded. "That's a long way away for me."

"No, it was long before that," he informed me. "Our oldest son was in middle school, and one day, he started hassling me that I was always tired, always grumpy, never did anything with them."

"Sounds familiar," I said. "Although I think David's given up on me already, and he's only five."

Jim nodded with a sympathetic grin.

"And I was so taken aback that he stood up to me like that," he continued. I was really overwhelmed with guilt, and work, and everything."

"I hear you," I concurred. "But what could you do?"

"Jamie, that's our oldest, said to me, 'Dad, do one thing with us this weekend where <u>you</u> have fun too'."

Jim looked at me, and then he continued.

"Just one thing. And I did," he said. "We all went on a hike in the woods. Vanessa and the kids packed a picnic. I was pretty overweight at the time, and I felt like crap, but I did it."

I nodded politely.

"I know what it's like to feel like your life is out of your control, Alex," he added pointedly.

Now he had my attention.

"It's just that, it's not that easy for me to pick up and take Joan and David for a hike, and everything is suddenly peachy," I admitted. "They're so used to me not being around, and," I trailed off.

"Everything starts with one small step," Jim said.

"Yeah," I agreed half-heartedly.

"If you're unhappy with your work, your family life, health, the way you feel, you're not helpless," he added. "You can change it. Think of the person with feelings of depression, who can't get out of bed to start their day. It's not like their legs don't work. The thing is, they don't need to think about the whole day. All they need to do is think about the one act of getting out of bed. That's the start."

I nodded to Jim with raised eyebrows. (Talk about mixed body language.)

He laughed. "Let me guess," he started. "You tried to make changes before."

Bingo.

"You know what it's like," I said.

"Oh yes," he finished. "You decide you're going to eat better, to exercise, to spend more time with the family, save more money, and then you have a crazy week at work and it all falls in the ditch."

"Pretty much," I agreed. "I've tried to get healthy, eat better, work out. A few times. Then you pull a few late nights, grab a little too much takeout, and you're off the treadmill."

"After a while, you stop trying," Jim concurred.

CHAPTER 14

I don't know how long we had been walking at this point, but I didn't check my watch for the first time in a long time.

Just walking felt great.

We didn't talk for a moment. Usually I would be scrambling to fill a silence gap, but this time I didn't.

"Anyway," Jim said comfortably. (I could tell he was trying not to lecture me.) "I had a few false starts, got frustrated and gave up a few times."

We were back to where we started. Jim looked at his watch. "Do you have time to walk a little more, or do you need to get back?"

I took a deep breath. This was the most relaxed I had been, between work hours, in a while.

"Yeah, I can stretch out lunch for once," I said. "So, what happened to change things?"

"I wish I could say that I had some sort of epiphany after that hike, and really changed my lifestyle," he told me. "But I didn't. I would try to cut back on work, be active with the family, the whole bit. Then work would creep up, I was always worried about money, keeping up with the Joneses, the whole deal. Jamie kind of gave up on me, and our two younger kids followed suit."

I nodded. "But obviously you flipped a switch at some point. What made it happen?"

"A couple of things actually," Jim said. "Two of my colleagues got sick. One had a heart attack, but bounced back. The other, Ted, had been a friend and a mentor. Work was his life. He was diagnosed with cancer. His kids were a little older than mine, but we had socialized with them as a family. He never took care of himself, and certainly never went to the doctor, so they caught it really late."

Jim took a deep breath, sort of a sigh.

"You don't have to tell me about it," I led.

"No, it's okay," Jim said. He took a breath. "Ted died within two months of the diagnosis."

"Oh, wow," I said sympathetically.

"The thing that got me was seeing his kids at the funeral," Jim continued. "They were solemn, but they didn't look sad."

I looked at Jim, my interest piqued.

"I mentioned that to Jamie the day after the funeral," Jim said. "He had great kids, so it really bothered me."

Jim shook his head.

"Jamie looked at me with spite in his eyes. He said, 'What do you expect, Dad? How can you miss someone who was never there to begin with?' Then he just walked away."

"Wow, harsh," I commented.

Jim looked at me and nodded. It was obvious this still got to him.

"The really harsh thing, was that Jamie was, at that moment, talking about me. Honestly, it was one of the saddest moments of my life. It was the game changer."

Soon, we were back at our starting point again. Jim gathered up the backpack. He looked at his watch, which made me look at mine.

"You probably need to get back," he said.

I nodded and we started walking.

"So, hold it," I said. "What did you do? Just quit your job and do something else? I mean, not everyone could or would do that."

"No, I didn't quit. I sat down with Vanessa that night," Jim finished. "Like I said, she had given up on me too, but I was really shaken after Jamie's comment. We had a long talk about all the important stuff. Health, family, lifestyle. She supported me. Later, we sat down with the kids, and we moved forward together, starting with small changes at first. I set limits for work, and, to tell the truth, I ended up being more productive while I was there."

"That's good Vanessa was so understanding. Joan and I have talked about getting in shape and eating healthy before," I told Jim. "It's never worked."

"I had some hiccups at first," Jim told me. "Most people do."

We were almost back at my building. I glanced up at it. I could feel my heart rate start to rev again.

"Whew," I commented. "I admire you. It's an amazing transformation."

Jim laughed good-naturedly.

"Thanks," he said. "The amazing thing to me was how simple it all was, once I burst through that bubble of feeling hopeless. Not that it was always easy. But once I realized I had control over my life and my habits, everything got better."

I shook Jim's hand. "Well, that was the most enlightening lunch I've had in a long time!"

He grinned self-consciously. "Hopefully I didn't sound too preachy, Alex," he said. "If I did, my apologies!"

"Not at all," I reassured him. "Lots of food for thought."

Jim looked up at my building. "I'd better let you get back to it," he said genially. "Thanks for sharing your lunchtime with me."

"I should be thanking you," I laughed. "I really appreciate it, Jim. Thanks again."

We both turned to go.

Then I turned back.

"Hey, Jim," I started.

He faced me. "Yeah," he said breezily.

"Want to meet for lunch next week?" I asked, a little awkwardly. "Another walk and talk? I'll bring the sandwiches."

"Sure! Sounds great, Alex."

And with a grin and a wave, he was off.

I looked up at my building again. It looked grayer and more imposing than usual, but the sky was a brilliant blue above it. With a deep breath, I started back.

CHAPTER 15

As I walked into my building, one of the senior partners in my company was rushing in behind me.

As we got to the elevator, he asked, "Alex, is it? How are you?"

"Yes sir, fine thanks. How are you?"

"Was that James Chipman you were speaking with?"

"Jim? He's my neighbor," I started.

The elevator dinged and the doors opened, obviously on his stop.

He raised his eyebrows and nodded at me.

Was it me or did he look impressed? I didn't get a chance to follow up. He dashed out of the elevator with a quick, "Have a good one!"

When I stepped off the elevator, onto my floor, my mind was all over the place. I had a lot of work to do, but I was really distracted by a lot of what Jim had said.

It was funny: After talking to him, I felt lighter than I had felt in a long time. At the same time, I felt like I had a rock in the pit of my stomach.

Bryan walked by, as I headed to my office.

"Hey buddy," he greeted me. "We missed you at lunch today! Taco Tuesday, man." I noticed he was rubbing his chest.

I didn't miss the heartburn that I usually got on 'Taco Tuesday'.

"Oh, yeah. Sorry to miss it," I told him. (I wasn't.) "I went for a walk in the park with a neighbor."

"What? Don't go getting all health nutty on us now," he laughed.

I nodded and laughed too. "No worries," I said.

"We were talking about the new tech company downtown," he followed. "They're already talking about expansion. Will is reaching out to them, to see if they need some guidance"

I felt a stab of stress. In this business, you had to be on top of everything. Missed information was a missed opportunity.

Bryan shrugged at me and walked off, taking a deep breath, and rubbing his chest again.

Bryan was probably my closest ally at work, and he had helped me a lot. I knew one thing though, looking at him walk off. I didn't want what he had.

CHAPTER 16

That evening, I made an effort to get home a little earlier.

When I walked in, it was business as usual: Joan and David in front of the TV, barely acknowledging my presence. They had already eaten. I guess I wasn't home that early after all.

I thought about what Jim had said, about his family giving up on him.

That night, as David was brushing his teeth, I asked Joan if we could just sit and talk for a while after David went to bed.

I needed her support. And frankly, besides the fact that Joan and I had almost zero quality time these days, she had also let herself go. She rarely worked out anymore. She had gained a few pounds, was eating like crap, having more to drink in the evenings, and just didn't have that spark she used to. Besides her time with David, she didn't look happy.

Joan had looked at me with a questioning expression on her face. "Sure," she said tersely.

I kissed David goodnight, but Joan always spends an extra few minutes with him, after they finish reading and before he goes to sleep.

I went into the family room and looked at some of our books on the shelves. I pulled out a couple of our old photo albums and sat down with them.

Joan has always taken lots of pictures. She gets those photo books made now.

The first one I opened had pictures from when David was two years old. It seemed like yesterday. We were so tired but it was such an amazing time. I was more focused on my family and most days left my work at work.

I opened the other old photo album. It was from just after college. I had just started my first job.

As I flipped through, I looked at pictures of Joan and I in our first apartment. That place was so small, but we were so happy there. (I know that's cliché.) I flipped through so many pictures of us with our college friends.

It seemed like a different world, and I looked like a different person. I liked the guy in the pictures better.

Joan walked into the family room. She looked a little surprised to see me looking through albums.

She paused, then came over and sat down with me.

"Remember laptop dinners?" I asked.

She smiled. We used to invite our friends over for supper on weekends. We'd make a big pot of stew or chili or something, and everyone would bring salads, sides or dessert. We'd all sit around with our supper on our lap, because we only had a little table. Afterwards, we'd play Pictionary or charades, or just talk and laugh.

None of us had very much. We were all just starting out in our careers, but they were the best times. It's funny, it is so true that the more you have the more you want. I wish I was that naive again.

We flipped through a few more pages. Then Joan took a deep breath and faced me.

"What did you want to talk about?"

"I just wanted to talk," I told her defensively.

"About what?" she followed. "I mean, you barely get home before I'm asleep most nights, you're stressed all the time, and now you want to talk?"

Wow, how did I not notice how bad things had gotten between us?

"I had lunch with Jim today," I told her.

She raised her eyebrows.

"We had a great talk," I continued. "Did you know he used to be a management consultant also?"

She looked surprised, shaking her head.

"It made me realize something. I want to make some changes," I said.

Joan kind of sucked in her breath.

"I want to get healthy and have more time with you and David. Really make some positive changes," I went on. "I just need your help to do that."

Joan exhaled, and just kind of crumpled.

"Are you serious?" she asked.

I was a little taken aback by her reaction.

I tentatively put my hand on hers and held on. "Yeah, I really am this time. I realized that I've been the pits to be around these days. That's when I am around. I've been trying to provide, but I've been really absent. I miss you. And David."

She hugged me. Joan is usually a rock, but she was kind of fighting back tears. I didn't think this was that big a deal.

Obviously it was.

"I've been feeling like I've been losing you lately," she said. "I just didn't know what you were going to say, when you said you wanted to talk."

I patted her hair as she went on. "I didn't know if you'd say you were sick, or you wanted out, or…"

I stopped her. "What? Out of this family? Are you kidding? You guys are everything to me."

She sighed and shook her head.

"Things will be different from now on," I promised. "I finally got it through my thick head that I can't take care of anyone else unless I take care of myself. I just need your support. We can make some changes together."

Joanie hugged me.

I felt better already.

CHAPTER 17

It's funny. After a long time of working my ass off and going through the motions at home like a zombie, I suddenly had two really strong feelings.

For one thing, I felt bad – guilty really – that Joan had thought I wanted out. I seriously hadn't realized how much I had checked out of our lives.

But on top of that was an overwhelming sense of optimism and positivity. Just the idea of taking control of my life again was exhilarating. I had been in such a rut, and I didn't want to feel this way anymore.

It just took someone (Jim) to make me stop and realize that I wasn't hopeless.

Sure, I'd had some failures in the past. But I was no dummy – I could learn from them. Just that difference in attitude made me feel so much happier and in control.

As I sat with Joan, it was like we were in a new relationship, with new opportunities.

It was awesome.

Joanie made a little pot of tea and we stayed up for a while longer, talking about what kind of changes we wanted to make, and what type of lifestyle we wanted. I wanted to have a vision for a healthier, happier life.

But I knew I wouldn't be able to just start coming home at five o'clock every day, and playing catch in the yard with David before our super healthy dinner.

If this was going to work, my changes and our changes had to be reasonable and achievable. At least, starting out.

It's like in business, when we do feasibility studies, to see if a new venture will work out. I didn't want to bite off more than I could chew.

We made a list of the most important things we wanted to change:

1. reign in the work hours
2. more family time, preferably active (not just watching TV)
3. eat better
4. get fit again
5. talk to each other when there's a problem, and work it out

Okay, that seemed like a lot at once, but Joan and I were on the same page. I, and we, were not going to change overnight. There would be some missteps, and that would be okay. If we got off track, we would get right back on.

Honestly, I was really proud of myself for this approach. I'd seen enough guys at work make New Year's resolutions or generally try to get healthy, just to crash and burn.

I texted Jim to thank him again for lunch, and touch base on next week. We'd meet again on Tuesday. I was hoping this would become a routine thing. No one had inspired me this much since my high school basketball coach.

That night, I don't know if it was the chamomile tea or the new outlook on life, or taking first steps, or that Joan and I went to bed together for the first time in a long time. I slept better than I had in ages.

CHAPTER 18

The next morning, I had breakfast with Joanie and David, before heading to work.

David was actually surprised when I asked him what he wanted for breakfast. He looked at Joan, questioningly.

"I'm going to have breakfast with you a little more often, buddy," I boomed. "What can I make you?"

David went to the fridge and got out the juice carton. "It's okay, Dad," he said in his little voice. "Mom always gets my cereal."

"Want me to get your juice?" I asked.

"Nah, that's okay," he said. He grabbed a glass. He wasn't used to me being around, and it was sad to think it felt strange to him.

He poured his juice, managing to get it all in the little glass, and took it to the table. Then he sat down and looked at me.

"Hot or cold cereal this morning, sweetie?" Joanie asked.

"Hot please, Mom," he said seriously.

He picked up the comics section of the newspaper.

Man, he was so cute.

I used to be really good with kids. I coached a mini basketball league when I was in college, with a couple of buddies. Now, it seemed normal to have my own son look at me awkwardly.

I brought my coffee over. "Anything good in the comics?" I asked.

He took a sip of his juice and shrugged. "I'll let you know."

I grinned at Joan with raised eyebrows. She winked.

I picked up the sports section and made another attempt. "How was soccer last night?"

"Goo-ood," he said. Joanie put his oatmeal in front of him.

"Yeah?" I looked at him.

He looked back at me, as if he was wondering whether he should engage.

Then, finally: "I scored a goal."

"Yeah? That's awesome buddy!" I high-fived him.

"Almost everyone else did, too."

We laughed. "Well that's okay," I started.

Joanie put some muffins on the table.

"David had an awesome kick." She looked at him. "It was a great goal, bud." Then she looked at me. "They gave everyone a chance at the end to try to score, but David's was in the middle of the game."

I patted his shoulder and he smiled.

I pointed to a comic strip in the paper. "Hey, I used to love this one," I said.

"Yeah, it's pretty good, but this one's my favorite," David replied.

"Want me to read it to you?" Joan asked.

"Dad can, if he wants," David told her.

It was the smallest gesture, but I can't tell you how good it made me feel.

I don't know if it was the fact that I skipped the greasy drive-thru breakfast sandwich and crappy coffee, or that I let myself enjoy the start of the day with my wife and kid; either way, I felt pretty good walking into the office.

That changed within thirty seconds of walking off the elevator.

"Whoa, somebody need to catch up on his beauty sleep?"

Yes, it was Bryan, walking up to me, looking at his watch.

I wasn't going to let him spoil my mood.

"Just having breakfast with my family," I shot back, in a positive tone.

"Ooh, how positively 'Leave It to Beaver' of you," he mocked, a little sharply.

I shrugged at him as I headed into my office. "Yeah well…" I trailed off.

How do you respond to that? I was still in the office by eight o'clock. I felt a little stress seep in.

No, I was not going to feel guilty about having breakfast with my wife and kid.

I started up my computer and zipped through some emails, then did a little research and got in touch with a couple of clients.

By 10:30, when I stepped into the staffroom to grab a coffee, I was feeling pretty good, better than I had felt at work in a while. I had just been more efficient in two and a half hours than I usually am each morning.

Bryan stepped in to grab a coffee. "Hey, a couple of us are going to grab some wings at twelve," he said. "Unless you're going to go home and have lunch and naptime," he teased.

"Bryan, what's the big deal," I said, a little miffed.

He slapped me on the back. "I'm just kidding, Alex. Don't be so sensitive."

He grabbed his black coffee and strode out, chuckling. "Just keeping you sharp, my man," he joked over his shoulder.

I stirred my coffee and put the milk back in the fridge, wondering how good a friend Bryan really was.

CHAPTER 19

I did join Bryan, Will, and a couple of others for wings at lunchtime.

You really did feel like you were missing out when you didn't socialize with the group. There was always at least one interesting tidbit of business information or gossip.

Plus, as much as I was miffed at Bryan this morning, he is a really funny guy with a heart of gold. He's given me tips, introduced me to the right people, and generally helped me in more ways than I could list.

As we finished off our lunch, I promised myself I'd cut back on the crappy food. Maybe next time I had lunch with the guys, I'd get a salad or some other healthy thing. Yes, I would risk mockery from Bryan, but I could take it.

I leaned over to Will. "We'd love to have you and Ashley over for dinner soon," I said. "We can show you our new house."

"That would be great," he bounced back.

"Super. Maybe just something casual," I followed. "I can barbeque."

Bryan was finishing up his conversation with one of the other guys at the table. Will and I instinctively stopped talking about social plans. He just nodded and flashed me a thumb's up.

The last time we invited Will and his wife, and Bryan for dinner, he brought (and I'll use Joan's words) 'a skanky ding-a-ling'. Then he proceeded to drink too much and turn into an asshole.

Well, maybe it wasn't that bad.

Yes, it was.

I think the turning point for Joan was when Star (yes, that was her real name) started talking about her favorite television shows, and listed 'Sponge Bob Square Pants' as one of her favorites.

"It's so funny," she had told Joan. "It's, like, a total commentary on society today."

"Oh yeah?" Joan had said gamely. "How?"

That had obviously confused Star.

The neat thing with Joanie (and something I had forgotten about her these days) is that she can talk to pretty much anyone. And she sees something positive in everyone. (Which obviously had included me lately.)

But she has no time for women playing dumb. Plus the fact that, as Bryan got more obnoxious, Star just giggled more.

Needless to say, we wouldn't add Bryan and his date of the week to the mix this time.

We finished up and started walking back to the office. I chatted with Will and one of the other guys, Sanjay, that we work with.

"What do you guys do to work out these days?" I asked.

"Actually, I just put in a home gym in our basement, a few months ago," Sanjay piped up.

"Oh yeah?" I perked up. "How do you like it?"

"It was great for about a month," he laughed. "Now my bench makes a pretty good laundry rack."

We laughed.

"No, but seriously, I try to make myself use it a couple of times a week," Sanjay said. "I just don't have a lot of time to go to a gym, so it's convenient."

I patted my stomach. "I've got to start working out again," I told them.

"I remember you played a lot of basketball when we were in school," Will commented.

"Yeah, I loved it," I told him. "But I've got to find something I can do on my own schedule. It can't be another thing I have to get to."

The guys nodded.

Bryan and the others had perked up to our conversation.

"The other thing," Sanjay said, "is that we have a TV in our basement, so it's less boring. Plus, my wife gets workout DVDs. She's all into Zumba these days, but she mixes it up."

"Ashley has some workout DVDs," Will added. "They're tough."

"Have you tried them?" I asked Sanjay.

"Honestly, yes. They're a good workout, and you don't have to think," he said, before turning to Bryan. "Okay Bryan," he laughed. "I can see you're dying to say something."

Bryan cocked his head back, seemingly appalled. "What? Sanjay, I was just thinking that now I know what to get you for your next birthday. Some workout gear."

"Oh, sorry Bry, that was nice of you," Sanjay bounced back.

"Now, what color leg warmers might match your outfits," Bryan jokingly thought out loud.

We all laughed.

But I still had to find something. I was determined to go forward with some healthy changes, and getting in shape was going to have to be a part of that.

CHAPTER 20

The next couple of days flew by. Besides a little flack from Bryan, and a few glances from my boss, work went pretty smoothly.

After talking to Jim, and for the first time in a while, I felt optimistic. I also felt like a donkey with someone holding a carrot so that I could just take the smallest nibble.

I had clarified what I wanted my life to be like. Now, would I be able to reach the whole carrot?

We spent the weekend doing odds and ends around the house.

I saw Jim as we were coming back from the hardware store, and he and Vanessa were heading out on foot. We all waved, David like crazy.

"Hi Jim and Vanessa!" That was David, who, I was realizing, really lets people know when he likes them.

"Hi there. Need a hand?" Vanessa called over, as we got out and opened the back of our SUV. They detoured toward us.

"Hi guys," Joanie said brightly. "Thanks, but I have two big strong guys with me, so we should be good."

At that, David flexed his little arm and looked at it.

Jim gave his arm a soft squeeze.

"Wow Vanessa, look at that bicep," Jim said, sounding impressed.

Vanessa rubbed his upper arm. "Oh my goodness David, you're very strong."

David puffed his chest out, then grabbed a bag from the back of the truck and started toward our front step. It wasn't heavy but it was a little awkward.

"Is that your new lamp?" Joanie asked as she rushed to catch the bag and open the door. "Be careful buddy."

She opened it and came back to where we were standing.

"That boy is the dictionary definition of adorable," Vanessa commented.

"Thanks," Joanie and I echoed each other.

"Where are you off to?" I asked.

"We're going to watch our oldest granddaughter dance," Jim said proudly. "Her dance school puts on a big spring show."

"She's a fantastic dancer," Vanessa added. "She does jazz and contemporary."

"Wow! Enjoy," Joan said, smiling.

"They're coming back here after for dinner," Jim said.

"Is that Jamie's daughter?"

"No, this is our youngest son, Andy, and his husband," Jim said proudly. "They have two little girls."

"Have fun" I said sincerely.

They both grinned. "We should get going, Vanessa," Jim said, taking her hand.

"Have a great afternoon," she said brightly, and they turned to go.

"Oh, and Jim," I said quickly.

He turned around.

"The weather's looking a little damp this week," I informed him. "I wonder if you just want to go to a restaurant? That is, if Tuesday is still good."

"Tuesday's great. Let's play it by ear with the weather," he told me. "We can always have a quick bite in an atrium and get outside after, if it's raining. I have umbrellas, even if it's just a quick bit of fresh air."

"Thanks for making the time," I started.

"I'm more than happy to," Jim said.

Later that evening, I glanced out the window and saw Jim and Vanessa with their son's family. Two little girls were doing cartwheels on the lawn. Jim, Vanessa, and two guys were sitting on the steps, a captivated audience. That must be Andy and his partner.

I thought of Jim's story about his oldest. Now they all seemed so close.

I was already looking forward to lunch.

The proverbial carrot felt like it was getting closer.

Or, more specifically, I felt like I was moving closer to it.

CHAPTER 21

The rest of the weekend flew by in a flurry of organizing and final touches on the house. It felt good to finally feel truly settled in.

The house felt warm and cozy. I liked that we had created a nice family space away from the tv, with books, games, and a comfy space to really veg out. Joanie bought these big square cushions that were a calming pale blue. David could sit right in the middle of them, with his legs crossed like a genie.

We ordered takeout, but not the old usual crap. We heard about this family-owned Greek restaurant, so we ordered healthy sample plates, with souvlaki, rice, Greek salad, pita bread and tzatziki. At first David was skeptical (as kids can be at that age), but he loved it.

I also talked to Joan again about work – hers and mine.

We had some clients coming in from out of town, and we were wining and dining them. Some work functions I could skip (and I would), but this would be mandatory.

Now that things were good between Joanie and me, I didn't want to mess up.

She, very astutely, had told me that she understood work was a priority. It just shouldn't be the only priority.

So, with that in mind, if I had a couple of late days or evenings out with work, I wanted to balance things at home.

She bought a calendar, one of those fill-in ones, and we promised each other we'd plan our weeks to include important activities for David, and family time.

Again, it was another simple, easy change.

Since this next couple of days was going to be busy with work, we'd plan a hike or some sort of extra time together on the weekend.

It was nice not to slink in after a late night, feeling guilty.

"Why don't we bring David to the Farmer's Market on Saturday morning," I suggested.

"That's a great idea," Joanie agreed. "A couple of people at work take their kids every weekend. I heard there's a little waffle stand. David would love that."

"Oh, and I mentioned to Will that we'd like to have them over soon," I added. "Would Saturday night work? We can make it early."

"Yeah, I'd love to see Ashley," Joanie smiled. "And Will, of course! No baby news yet?"

I shook my head.

"Okay, I'll cross that topic off the list," she said.

Then we talked about Joanie's job. In a nutshell, she hated it.

Joanie had done extremely well in business school, and was very savvy and well liked. But, early on, she had held a position that involved a lot of travel.

After David arrived, she took a year off, then she changed jobs to something that was more stable, with no travel.

As she said at the time, she got off the 'up escalator'.

Book authors and female business leaders will tell women to lean in, buck up, and go for it, but throw a few sleepless nights on top of important presentations, etc., and unless you have a live-in nanny who does housework, it's pretty tough.

Joanie's present job was a grind. She wasn't being challenged, she rushed David to pre-school, then rushed to pick him up from after school programming. She ended up feeling guilty and unhappy – a fact I only learned recently.

Speaking of guilty, I should have realized she wasn't happy, or at least asked her every once in a while.

We sat on the couch and talked about some solutions.

The thing Joanie really wanted to do was cut back her work hours, or at least be able to work from home sometimes. Now that David was going to be starting in grade primary, she wanted to be able to have a little more time with him after school, or to volunteer with his class.

We weren't living the life of luxury, but we were lucky, in that we could afford for Joanie not to work full-time. But some of the best positions in the business world were all or nothing.

Really, I think Joanie needed to know it was okay to make a change, in a year that we had already had a major one (the house).

But sometimes you have to shake things up. I already felt so good about my new attitude toward life, I agreed that a change would be good for Joanie.

"I'm just going to put my feelers out," she told me. "See what's out there these days."

"That's a great idea," I agreed. "Maybe connect with a few of our old business school friends, and chat with them."

"I might call Lydia and invite her out for lunch," she thought out loud.

(Lydia was a year ahead of us in college, and one of Joanie's mentors. In school, she was a public relations whiz.)

"What's she doing these days?" I asked.

"She was the head of a women's business initiative," Joanie answered. "She has lots of connections."

"That's great," I said, rubbing her shoulder.

"Plus, I'd love to catch up with her," Joanie followed, with a glint in her eye.

I loved seeing her look excited about something again. As much as Joanie wanted better, more flexible work hours, she also wanted to feel excited about what she was doing. Neither of us had realized what a rut we had been in.

Talking about what kind of vision we had for our lives, and what was important to us was the simplest thing in the world – and the most essential first step.

CHAPTER 22

The next couple of days flew by as quickly as the ones before.

When Tuesday rolled around, the weather looked like it would hold. I met Jim at the park. He was chatting with a pretty stately looking fellow as I walked up.

Jim waved at me, and the other guy shook his hand and patted him on the shoulder before walking briskly off.

"Good to see you, Chip," the man called, waving.

"Let's all get together soon," Jim called back.

"Hey Jim," I greeted him brightly. "Was I breaking up a conversation?"

"Not at all, just an old friend," he said cheerfully. "Chip?"

Jim laughed. "And an old nickname."

As I unpacked a large paper bag, I looked at Jim sheepishly.

"I went to the deli," I admitted.

"Ooh, that little place around the corner?" Jim asked, pointing back toward my building. "Mimi's place?"

"Yeah," I laughed. "You know Mimi?"

"Are you kidding? Mimi was legendary when I was working," Jim laughed. "I've got to pop in sometime. I didn't think she was still there!"

"Oh yeah, Mimi's still a going concern," I nodded.

I had bought chopped veggie salads, a couple of Mediterranean wraps, and yogurt parfaits. I figured Jim wasn't a soda guy at all, so I had gotten a couple of waters and some sparkling juice.

"This looks great," Jim said enthusiastically.

"I've been trying to get less takeout," I told him as we started eating.

"I know what you mean, but if you make good choices in your takeout, it can be pretty healthy," Jim reminded me. "Like these Greek wraps. I forgot how good Mimi makes them."

"I know," I agreed between bites.

We settled into easy chitchat as we ate. Jim and I knew a few of the same people, and I caught him up on some of the downtown business gossip.

When we finished, he stretched. "Want to walk?" he asked.

"Definitely," I said as we started to pack up the remains of lunch.

"Thanks for lunch, Alex," Jim started.

"Thank you," I cut in. "I really appreciate your perspective on things, Jim. In fact, I'd love to meet for lunch any time you feel like it."

I had realized that every time I spoke with or interacted with Jim, I felt better.

When I thought of how negative I had been when I first met Jim, I felt bad. He had really opened up my eyes. He had become not just a mentor, but a friend.

"Absolutely," Jim agreed. "Anytime."

'Anytime' became once a week. As we walked on that day, we talked about some pretty simple stuff, mainly lunch, food, how it can make you feel energized and ready to go, or make you feel like crap.

Jim was not a preachy guy, and he had been there, sitting in business dinners, etc. (At least, from what I could gather. He wasn't one to give details about his former work life!)

He was all about starting with moderate, attainable changes, and going from there.

He gave me some great tips for eating healthier at dinners. Stuff like ordering lower fat entrees, filling up on healthy salads, ordering sauces on the side, or substituting, and drinking more water.

Even at work, bringing healthy, easy snacks so I didn't hit the wall at 3pm and run out for coffee and a sugary snack.

A lot of these changes started at the grocery store or market.

That lunch with Jim was a welcome respite from a crazy week.

I would come to look forward to lunch with Jim every week as a breath of fresh air.

CHAPTER 23

That week, besides a heavy workload in the day, we were meeting our clients for drinks and dinners on back-to-back nights. The first night was Italian, followed by a high-end steak house the night after.

You can't take clients out for dinner, and then just order a salad and water. So, even though I wanted to eat healthier, it was starting slowly this week! I did skip a couple of high fat sauces, so that was a beginning!

Even though the dinners were officially work, our clients were a great bunch, and we had a lot of laughs.

Bryan, as leader in our section, is the ultimate host. He was ordering lobster appetizers for the table, and kept the food and drinks flowing. I don't want to know how many bottles of wine we went through during both dinners. We finished with scotch. Midway through the week, I felt like one of David's (over)stuffed animals.

All I could think about was getting to the weekend. My best intentions of starting to exercise were going to have to wait 'til another week.

By Thursday evening, when I got home (on time) for dinner, I was tired and sluggish.

Joanie had made a big salad with chicken, and gotten focaccia bread. We had water with a slice of lime in it, and David had a glass of milk. It was just what I needed after all the heavy food.

After having lunch with Jim, Joanie and I had decided to be more conscious of what we were buying. We decided to spend 20 minutes on Sunday morning discussing the week's meals and what was needed. Then we'd be off to the store with a focus. I found it really helped in making the smart choice.

Joanie had really made an effort to make meals healthier recently, as opposed to all the processed foods and takeout we had been eating before. I really appreciated it, and I think we all felt better.

We sat down to eat, and David started batting his food around his plate.

"I don't like this," David told us.

(Just the kind of positive reaction you want when you're trying to make a change! Luckily, Joanie had some kind of 'mom immunity' to David's criticisms.)

"Why not?" Joan asked.

"I hate salads," he stated.

"No you don't, sweetie," Joan corrected him.

"Yes I do. I hate them," he said, starting to get sulky.

"Well that's funny, because you liked salads last week," Joan said lightly. "Are you sure you're not an impostor," she joked.

"Yes," he said. "What's an impostor?"

Joanie has so much patience. The last thing I felt like doing was arguing with my kid over a bunch of cucumbers and tomatoes, but Joanie was keeping her cool.

"It's someone who pretends to be someone they're not," I said. "Mom's joking that you're an impostor, because the David we know really likes veggies and salads."

"Okay then, I'm a spy," David said, sitting back, "who hates salad."

Joanie and I looked at each other, trying to keep straight faces. You had to give him points for originality.

"I want mac and cheese," he followed, obstinately.

"Sweetie, I can't give you mac and cheese right now," Joanie told him. "But I'll make some cheesy noodles tomorrow for supper."

"No, now," David shouted. He shoved his plate toward the center of the table.

"Hey. That's enough," I said, a little louder than I meant to. He jumped. Joan gave me her 'look of wrath'.

Wow. David's usually a pretty laid back kid. I didn't know what had gotten into him, but frankly, I didn't have a lot of reserve patience. All I wanted to do was have a relaxing dinner with her and David.

Joanie put her hand up. "Buddy, I can separate your veggies and chicken into sections for you, but I can't make you something else tonight. Hand me your plate please."

David was sitting back in his chair, just looking angry at the world. But he picked up his plate and gave it to her, then he sat back and crossed his arms.

"I'm sorry for raising my voice buddy," I conceded.

"I forgive you, I guess," he said grudgingly.

When Joanie and I decided to have a kid, we always said we'd be really calm and open communicators. Which is why David wasn't surprised when I asked, "Why are you so grumpy tonight?"

"I'm not grumpy, you're grumpy," David shot back.

Joanie and I looked at each other, trying not to laugh. Boy, David was in a foul mood, but he was being so cute.

A few weeks ago, I would have just been miffed that he was being hard to get along with, because I was in a bad mood most of the time.

"Who did you play with today?" Joanie asked. I thought it was an odd segue, but whatever.

"Isaiah and Kevin," he said.

"Great," I said. "What did you do?"

"We chased Lily around," he told us glumly. "Then me and Isaiah went on the monkey bars."

"Isaiah and I," Joanie corrected.

"Why did you chase her?" I asked.

"Kevin wanted to," he said, with his own brand of kid disgust.

"Did she want you to chase her?" I asked.

"No. She's nice," he reported. "She was pretty mad."

"Yeah, I would be too," Joanie told him.

"Yeah. Isaiah and I wanted to go on the monkey bars, so I told Kevin I didn't want to play with him," David said solemnly. "And we said sorry to Lily."

"That's good," I led.

"Oh yeah. Lily gave Kevin a fat lip," he finished.

"Well," Joanie mused, "I think there are a couple of lessons in there that you realized. Treat everyone with respect. And don't follow what someone else is doing just because they tell you to."

"Yeah, and don't mess with Lily," David added.

"Good point," Joanie said, high-fiving David.

Later that night, when I had just finished reading to David, I said to him, "I'm glad you told us about Kevin today. It sounds like he's kind of a bad influence."

He looked up at me with his doe eyes and shrugged. "Yeah," he said simply. Then, "What's a bad influence?"

Trying not to laugh, I said, "It's when someone you know does stuff that they shouldn't do, and sometimes it makes you want to do those same things."

"Yeah, Kevin doesn't make good choices," he informed me.

"Wow, that's pretty mature of you to say," I told him.

"The teachers say it," he said, snuggling in and under the covers with his bear. I ruffled his hair.

Joanie popped in. "Goodnight George," she announced. (That's the bear.) David held George up for us to give him a kiss.

Then I gave David a kiss. "Goodnight little man," I said softly. "I love you."

"Love you too, Dad," David said, in his sweet, sleepy voice.

I got up as Joanie said goodnight to David, thinking about bad influences and good choices.

CHAPTER 24

Since I had started taking the stairs instead of the elevator, I saw a whole different group of people.

They were always pretty positive every morning. As I walked up the stairs at work the next morning, I felt pretty positive too, like I was making some good strides in my self-improvement.

Still, I couldn't wait for the weekend. Now that I was around a little more, and engaged at home, I realized what I had been missing. Joanie was happier, and we were getting along great. We were also way more affectionate toward each other. I felt like the spark was back in our relationship (a change I was very happy with)!

We've all jokingly said 'happy wife, happy life', but it wasn't just that. Since I had re-focused my priorities, we were connecting better.

David was a joy to hang out with, and I realized how much I had been missing before.

All this sounds like I just snapped my fingers and decided to make a change, and everything was peachy. It didn't happen that way.

Truth is, I was starting to get some flack at work. It was mainly joking around, but the message was clear: you haven't been working as hard as the rest of us.

Sure, I wasn't burning the midnight oil every night and coming in early every day; but I was clearer, more efficient, and I think I was doing a better job than six months ago. My numbers were showing it.

You can probably guess who was ribbing me the most: Bryan.

As I came out of the stairwell, I just about ran into him.

"Hey," I said. "Good morning!"

"Hey! What are you doing coming out of the stairwell? Is there a fire?" he asked.

I laughed. "I was coming to work," I said, choosing not to give a sarcastic answer.

"Why? Is the elevator broken?" he followed. (He was serious.)

We started walking down the hall, toward our offices.

"No," I told him, upbeat. "Sometimes I take the stairs. It's not that many floors."

"Wow, next you'll be coming in with a yoga mat," he snorted. He looked at his watch. "So you missed our chat about our new client," he said, trailing off.

"Was there a meeting scheduled that I didn't hear about?"

"Not an official meeting, but we got talking over coffee this morning, and Sanjay had some interesting approaches," he told me.

"Sanjay, the new guy?"

"Yeah, he's pretty sharp," Bryan said with a tone that was meant to sound casual, but there was an edge there. He patted my shoulder and walked off.

I walked into my office, feeling a little less pleased with myself, and thinking a little more about bad influences.

CHAPTER 25

During business school, a group of us used to go to the Saturday morning Farmer's Market. We'd buy bread and whatever was in season, and hang out over coffee and a cinnamon roll. There were always a couple of musicians playing.

I loved people watching. There was always a wide array of people, from college students to young families, yuppies, hipsters, and folks that were pretty hard-core about organic everything.

With the 'buy local' movement being even stronger these days, the market had turned into a thriving heart of the city on Saturdays.

After a long week, punctuated at the end with some mixed vibes from Bryan and my boss, I was glad to get back to the Market.

Joanie and I walked in, holding David's hand, and he didn't know which way to go first! I couldn't believe so much time had passed since we had been here.

"This is awesome," David said excitedly.

"Want to get a waffle?" Joanie asked him.

Needless to say, the answer was yes, and we got waffles with fresh fruit on them, and sat down to eat on the wide stairs that we used to sit on as students.

There was a little girl dancing in front of a duo playing fiddle and guitar.

"We should come here every week," David said.

"Yeah, I forgot how much fun it is here," Joanie said, giving him a squeeze.

"You used to come here?" David asked.

"Yeah, Daddy and I used to come and hang out with our friends when we were in school," Joanie told him.

"Like, my school?" David asked, incredulously.

Joanie wiped some blueberry off his nose and smiled. "When we were in college, buddy."

David nodded. He started clapping his hands to the music, and we sat for a few minutes more. Then I gave David a couple of bucks to toss into the musicians' case, and we cruised around the stalls to get fresh veggies and greens, barbeque stuff, gelato, some local eggs, and bread.

As we were just about to go, someone called out, "Hey Joanie, Alex!"

We turned around. It was Bridgette and Sam, a couple of our old classmates from business school.

There was a quick flurry of hugs and handshakes, along with "I can't believe it's been so long" and "You look great!"

I actually couldn't believe it had been so long. (And they did look great!)

We introduced David, whose little outstretched hand, all ready for a handshake, charmed them.

"Oh my gosh, we should get together and catch up," Bridgette said. She bent down to David's level. "We have a boy and a girl, right around your age."

David nodded seriously.

Then to us, "My folks are in town, so they're with them, around here somewhere."

"It's so great to see you both," Joanie replied. "We'd love that."

Joanie and Bridgette exchanged contact info, while I picked David up and talked to Sam.

"So David, has your dad got you shooting hoops yet?" Sam asked.

"No, not yet," David replied.

"He was a pretty good player in school," Sam commented, then tousled his hair.

"Work and everything got a little out of control," I told Sam. "But we bought a new house, and we're settling in."

Sam nodded like he could relate. "Where'd you buy?" he asked.

"In Lakewood, not too far from the park," I told him.

"Wow," he nodded. "You must be doing well!"

I waved it off. "We lucked into a really friendly neighborhood." (That was an understatement. Everyone was amazing and I felt like Jim was saving my life!)

Sam and Bridgette both looked pretty fit still. He had always been a good guy in school, and pretty clean living. We had played intramural basketball together. I didn't know how we had lost touch.

We talked about houses, work, and neighborhoods for a couple of minutes, but by then

David was getting antsy, and had had enough of the grownup talk.

With a promise to get together soon, we were off, loaded down with our veggies and other market stuff.

Somehow though, I felt lighter than I had in a while. After talking about trying to find balance, I finally felt like I was finding some – and it was awesome.

Those insane work hours and crappy meals weren't looking so attractive now.

CHAPTER 26

The rest of the day was great. We took David to the park, and ran into the Johnsons, the neighbors who had the barbeque. David had a great run around, and we shot a few hoops with Kim and Ty and their kids. (I can see why they played college hoops.)

On our way back, we ran into Jim and Vanessa. They were outside, gardening, happy as clams.

We chatted for a few minutes, and then Joanie excused herself, running in to get a few things ready for the barbeque. David followed her, but I hung back.

"I'm really appreciating your advice and perspective, when we have lunch, Jim," I told him.

"It's my pleasure, Alex," he said brightly. "How's everything been going?"

"Well, I'm finding some balance between work and home. I realize that it's all just life, and looking at it separately was giving me anxiety. I just need to get healthier now," I said, patting my stomach.

"You mean eat healthier?" he asked.

"We've been improving on that," I followed. "We even took your advice for the grocery store.

We're buying way less processed stuff. And I forgot how great the farmer's market is." I laughed. "But I meant fitter. I've got to get rid of this gut."

He perked up. "There's a nice neighborhood fitness center. Want to come with me tomorrow morning? I'm going around eight."

I thought for about two seconds. "You know what? I will join you."

"Fantastic! I'll meet you out front at eight. It's near the park, just a few minutes run," he informed me.

I flashed a thumb's up and smiled. I felt pretty grateful that Jim had taken me under his wing.

"See you then," I confirmed, as I headed toward our house.

I got a couple of things done around the house. And that evening, Will and Ashley came over for a barbeque.

CHAPTER 27

It felt like it had been a while since we had invited anyone over. These days, by the end of the week, the last thing either Joanie or I felt like doing was making the house look good, then shopping and cooking for extra people.

I know that sounds bad, but it was what everyone at my office thought too. By the end of the week, you just wanted to relax.

So, I had forgotten what a great feeling it was, and how energizing it is to gather with friends and share a meal.

Will and Ashley are really fun, down to earth people. Will and I had started to chat more at work, and we share a lot of the same values. Whenever Joanie and Ashley see each other, it's a gabfest.

They arrived just after five. Ash had made a salad and Will handed me a bottle of organic wine he had told me about. Ashley handed David a little bottle of sparkling juice, which was really thoughtful.

"Thank you, Ashley and Will," he recited.

"You're welcome, David," Ashley said sweetly. Then she gave him a little gift bag. He took it and pulled out a book.

Joanie bent down beside David and looked at the cover. "*Jigsaw Jones*," she read. "That looks great, David!"

"My nieces and nephews read the series. I wanted to see what you thought of it. It's about a boy in grade two, who's a really good detective," Ashley told him. "And he helps out all his friends."

David gave Ash a big hug. "Thank you so much, Ashley," he said sincerely.

You could feel how much Ashley wanted kids. I hoped it would happen for them soon.

We ushered them out to the back patio, and we had a drink. We had put a couple of large planters on the deck, and some comfortable chairs and a table.

Lately, we had put in a lot of time, cleaning up the garden and planting new things. I was proud of it, but we'd been enjoying doing it, as much as the finished product.

There's something about gardening that inherently makes you chill out. I don't know if it's digging in the soil, or the fact that you can turn your brain off, or starting something that will just grow… But getting work done in the garden was simple and pure enjoyment.

"Your yard looks fantastic," Ashley commented.

"Want to see my veggie garden?" David asked her.

"Heck yes," she bounced back.

David took her by the hand and led her to the side of the yard, toward the back, with his veggies.

We had planted them together, and David was in charge.

"Can I see them too?" Will asked.

"Yes! Come with me," David said proudly.

We all went over and David pointed out his zucchinis, peas, cucumbers, and strawberries.

"I'll give you some veggies once they're big, okay Ashley?" David told her seriously.

"Wow, thanks David," she said. "Maybe you could help me plant some veggies too."

He nodded and high-fived her.

We finished our drinks, and this delicious fresh salsa and chips that Joanie had made, and then I started the barbeque.

It was such a beautiful evening, so we decided to eat outside. I grilled chicken and we sliced them for burgers. Joanie had gotten guacamole, and made a lime cilantro sour cream. With the salads, it was a delicious meal.

David ate with us, then we excused him until dessert, because, in his words, "grown ups talk SO much."

And we did talk about a lot: old business school friends, new houses, vacations (or lack thereof, with new houses), and events going on in the city.

The one thing we tried to stay away from was work. Ashley works in public relations, but she just wanted to be home with a posse of kids. Joanie, while excited about the prospect of changing jobs, didn't want to say anything. And, for Will and I, there was an unspoken feeling that talking about work induced heartburn and other unsavory feelings these days.

Finally, work did come up, in the form of Bryan.

"I know he's supposed to be so successful," Ashley commented. "But he seems a little sad."

"How can you say that?" Will countered. "When we ran into him at the wine shop, he was just about walking on air."

"When was that?" I asked.

"This morning," Will nodded. "He asked what we were up to this weekend."

"And I told him we were catching up with old friends," Ash interrupted. "I left names out of it."

"Thank you!" That was Joanie.

Ash nodded to her knowingly. Obviously they shared the same feeling about Bryan.

Ashley continued. "He went on about his epic weekend. He had just dropped his kids back at his ex-wife's place, and was going to binge watch some TV show, then get some ribs from the new southern barbeque place on Queen Street. Then meet up with some buddies downtown. He was buying a bunch of imported beer."

She paused for a moment. "If that's what turns your crank, go for it; but it just sounded kind of sad to me. He'll be hungover for most of tomorrow."

"That's the thing with Bryan," I commented. "He works like a crazy man all week, then he either parties or does nothing."

"And then on Monday, he lets everyone know how awesome he is and how lame everyone else is," Will added.

"I think he's always trying to play up how awesome his life is, but it seems a little empty to me," Ashley said.

I hadn't thought of it that way before, but that was so true. It obviously got under Will's skin too.

"The guy has no balance. It's all or nothing," Will said derisively.

Will had hit the nail on the head. It was all about balance.

We all were sitting back in our seats at the table now. The sunny day was becoming a calm, warm evening.

"It's too bad," Will spoke up. "Bryan is a brilliant guy."

"And a really nice guy," I added.

"Oh yeah, he'd give you the shirt off his back," Will agreed. "Unfortunately, now that shirt would be beer soaked, wing stained, and smelling like a college frat party. And a little bit of sadness."

There was a pause, then we all started laughing.

"You should write, sweetie," Ashley told him half-mockingly. "You've got a flare for drama."

"Yeah, screw the financial world," Joanie added.

Will laughed too. "I've got to stop talking about work. It bums me out on the weekend. I'll either write the next great tragedy or I'll have a heart attack."

CHAPTER 28

A little later, we got up and took another look at the yard. It was nice to get up. I found lately that sitting for a long time at work or at a dinner was getting tougher to handle. Or maybe I was just noticing it more. I had to move.

David came out with his soccer ball and was dribbling it around, showing off a little the way kids that age do.

I caught a glance at Ty and Kim walking by out front. I waved and they waved back. "How are you?" I asked, as they came toward the gate.

"Hey guys," Ty shot back, upbeat. "Just rounding up our kids."

Three heads popped up. "Hi," they chorused. Kim laughed.

"Hey," Joanie said warmly. "Come and meet our friends."

"Hi guys!" David was pumped. I think we were starting to bore him.

They came in and introductions were made. The kids instantly started goofing around with the soccer ball, and we invited them all for dessert.

"We don't want to interrupt," Kim said, as we motioned them in.

"And don't worry about anything for the kids. They're happy to play," she added.

"Are you kidding? We'd love to have you join us. I have these great fruit puree popsicles that they can have, and we have a really refreshing sorbet for us," Joanie told Kim.

Joan, Ashley, and Kim went in the house, while the rest of us supervised the kids. (Okay, we hung out.)

When Kim and Ty's oldest called out, "Kids against dads," we joined in, setting up makeshift goals.

It was fun (and funny), and it reminded me that I really needed to get in shape!

The girls had obviously gotten distracted inside, but when they came out, the kids sat on the grass and had those fruit-sicles and we had a raspberry gelato and lime sorbet. Joan had also made some neat oatmeal and apple cookies, and everyone grabbed a couple.

A little later, we sat around on the deck as the kids played and looked for fireflies in the yard.

We all had a mug of coffee or herbal tea, and conversation was easy. It's interesting how you can bring together two sets of friends, and everyone clicks.

I learned a few things about Kim and Ty. I knew Ty was a family doctor, but I didn't know that Kim had been an athletic therapist.

"Your kids are awesome," Ashley told Kim and Ty.

"Thanks," Ty said. "They're a lot of fun. And, by the way, you're seeing their best behavior."

Kim laughed. "True that, baby."

"Do you have kids?" Ty asked.

"Not yet, but we're hoping soon," Ashley answered sincerely. "We're more than ready."

"So you still know what sleep is," Kim joked.

"Any advice?" Ashley followed. "I mean, how do some couples get pregnant so easily, and others have such a hard time?"

"Well, there are a lot of factors. But I'll tell you one thing. Have fun," Ty answered.

We all laughed. Will high-fived Ty.

Ty laughed. "No, seriously though. Don't let yourself get too stressed about it."

"The only thing that stresses most guys is that they don't get enough," Joanie joked.

We all laughed, but then Ty added, "You don't even want to hear some of the lengths couple go through to get pregnant. And positions."

"Seriously?" I asked, amid the laughter.

"I've had guys come in and beg me to tell their wives to lay off," Ty said, nodding.

"Wow," Joanie said.

"Please let's get to that point," Will implored Ashley, jokingly.

We all laughed.

"Us too," I said, mock-sincerely to Joanie.

"Uh, we're not trying to have another baby," Joanie shot back.

"Oh, right," I said, snapping my fingers.

We all laughed and segued into another subject.

But it hit me. Stress really affected every aspect of our lives if we let it.

CHAPTER 29

We wound down a little while later, after more easy conversation and a lot of laughs.

I spent so much time in forced social settings for work, I had forgotten how much fun it is to get friends together and have everything click.

After we tucked David in, Joanie and I tidied up the last of the dishes. Since we hadn't entertained in a while, we had specifically kept everything easy, so we wouldn't be up late washing dishes.

We both loved this part of an evening with friends: talking about funny moments, bits of gossip, and other little things.

"We should have Will and Ashley over again with Ty and Kim," Joanie suggested.

"Yeah, they all really hit it off," I agreed, putting the leftover cookies in a container. "Did you see Ash blush when Ty was talking about couples trying to get pregnant?"

Joanie whipped her dish towel over her shoulder and turned to me. "I know! She was laughing about it, but she told me earlier that she tried this new yoga pose to, uh, increase their chances of getting pregnant!"

"Yoga pose?"

"Okay, maybe not yoga, but she was doing some kind of shoulder stand thing," Joanie said, trying not to laugh.

She shook her head. "I don't mean to laugh," she said. "Ash is trying to seem casual, but she's borderline stressed. Maybe Ty's comment will help her chill out."

"Yeah, Will's in that happy stage of lots of nookie right now, but he made an offhand remark last week at work about feeling like a prize stud. They're so great together. I hope they don't let this get to them."

"Easy for us to say," Joanie said.

I nodded. "Good point."

We stood at the sink, with Joanie washing a few serving dishes and me drying.

"Speaking of great, it is so nice to see you getting back to yourself," Joanie said sincerely. "Not to diss anyone, but I was relieved to hear you and Will separating yourselves a little bit from Bryan."

"Yeah, I've always felt a certain loyalty to him," I started.

"I know."

"But he's pretty self-destructive in a lot of ways. It took me a while to realize it," I told Joanie.

"And I get that you have to do the social thing with him at work," Joanie added.

"Yeah. And he has helped me out a lot," I said.

"I understand. But I'm glad you can separate him being a mentor in business, to him being someone you want to hang out with or emulate," Joanie said, bringing home the thought that was on my mind.

I nodded. It was true. Bryan was a good guy with a big heart. But I didn't want to be like him.

"I missed you," Joanie led, kissing me. "Glad you're back."

"Me too," I said, kissing her back.

And with that, clean up was over.

CHAPTER 30

The next morning, nice and early, I got up with David, who was bright as a chipmunk. I got out our mini-blender to make a smoothie.

David helped me, picking out the flavor (blueberries and banana), and we sat on the back patio with our morning drinks.

"That was fun last night," David said as he took a loud and slurpy sip. (I had to stifle a laugh, it was so cute.)

"Yeah, your mom and I were saying that we'd like to get together with friends a little more often," I agreed. "Your friends too."

Another loud sip. "I agree, Dad. Having friends makes you feel happy."

I smiled at David and nodded. It was so true. And suddenly a thought hit me. Sitting there with him, looking at the bluish smoothy on his top lip, I realized how fast the time was going to fly. I would turn around and he'd be grown up.

I gave him a kiss on the head.

"Why'd you kiss me, Dad?" Another slurp.

"Because I love you buddy," I answered.

He got up with his smoothie still in his hands and gave me a (wet) kiss on top of my head. "I love you too Dad."

As he sat back down, I had an almost desperate need to stay on track, to be healthy, and to savor time with my family in particular, and friends.

We hung out for a bit longer, watching the birds in the yard, and talking about our garden. But it was almost eight and he wanted to snuggle with Joanie, who was having a little sleep in.

He grabbed a book and I got ready to go.

At eight o'clock on the dot, I stepped outside.

There was Jim.

"Good morning," he called to me, in his usual chipper tone.

"Hey Jim," I said (more brightly than I meant to).

"You sound upbeat," Jim commented, as we started down the street. "How's your weekend been so far?"

"We had some friends for dinner last night, for the first time in a while," I recounted. "Kim and Ty and their kids stopped over and joined us. It was a lot of fun."

"They're a great family," Jim agreed.

He sped up and looked at me questioningly.

I nodded and we eased into an easy run. "This okay?"

"When we used to have people over, we would clean and cook all day, have some big meal, drink too much, stay up too late, and feel like crap the next day," I told Jim. "But we started early, did a an easy healthy meal, and didn't drink too much. I feel great."

"I know what you mean," Jim said. "It's nice to hang out with friends, but not pay for it before and after."

"Exactly." It hit me again: Jim was a cool guy.

We were running smoothly and not too fast, but I was getting a little winded.

"Let's walk for a minute," Jim suggested.

I was happy to.

"A friend who used to coach varsity track at the university gave me some great advice," Jim started. "Whenever his athletes were injured and not able to run for a while, he would start them back on a walk-run program, just to ease into it."

"Really?" (Sounded good to me about now!) "Competitive runners?"

"Yeah, and lots of them were national caliber runners. But he said not jumping into the hard stuff right away was better for the body, and the mind."

"That makes sense."

Jim laughed. "With his runners, he said it got them hungry to get back in shape. They hated the walking part. I like it though."

We eased into a run again. And then we were at the fitness center.

It looked pretty new from the outside.

We walked in. It was a colorful, airy space. There at the desk was a girl who looked like a college student.

"Hi Megan," Jim said warmly.

"Hey, good morning Jim," she shot back. "How are you?"

I was really getting the sense that everyone loved this guy.

"Wonderful, thanks," he smiled. "Megan, this is my friend Alex. They just moved into our neighborhood a while ago. He's going to use one of my passes."

"Absolutely," Megan said, smiling at me. "Welcome, Alex."

In business school, we did a case study on fitness chains and workout places, so I knew about having fit, good-looking people as staff, and the super friendly 'we love you' approach. But it was still nice. I understood why that's so successful.

"Jim's an awesome guide," Megan said, but if you have any questions, I'm happy to help. Or just ask any of our staff. Everyone's super here."

"Thanks Megan," I smiled back.

"Oh, Megan, Vanessa said to say thanks a lot for that cookie recipe," Jim added.

"Did she make them?" Megan asked.

"Yes, and we loved them. Our grandkids went crazy over them too," Jim laughed. "They were awesome."

Jim turned to me. "Megan gave Vanessa this energy bar recipe, but you make them like cookies. Just super."

"Mm, sounds good," I commented.

We walked past the turnstiles.

"What do you feel like doing?" Jim asked me. "There's a cardio room, free weights, TRX, some machines," he trailed off.

I used to go to the gym with the guys in college, and it was pretty much free weights, so I chose that. The thought of getting myself tangled up in one of those strength machines wasn't very appealing.

We walked into an area with benches and weights, but also a lot of mats, stability balls, kettle bells, and some other weighted balls.

Again, there were light walls and an organized set up. It was clean and bright, as opposed to dingy. That made it so much more inviting to work out.

A few people were there who seemed like regulars. A few of them greeted Jim or said hi to both of us.

I nodded at Jim, and with an, "Okay," I was off toward the bench press.

"Do you need a spot?" he called after me.

"No thanks. I'm going to start easy," I grinned. "Like your coach friend says."

Jim headed to a mat and did a couple of stretches. He rolled over some kind of soft cylinder, like he was stretching out his back.

A little while later, after I had done a few sets of bench press, leg press, and some other exercises from my old repertoire, I went over to where Jim was doing some exercise with a stability ball. He had his hands on a mat and his feet on the ball, rolling the ball in different directions.

"Wow Jim," I commented. "That's impressive."

He finished and got off the ball effortlessly. "Yeah, it's great for your core," he told me. "I like a lot of these exercises."

It had been a long time since I had worked out, and I always went back to the same old thing, so I was intrigued.

"Where did you learn them?" I asked.

"Vanessa got me a few sessions with a personal trainer as a gift last year, and he showed me a lot of these. They've got a couple of good trainers here, if you ever want to learn some new tricks," he pumped.

I was already feeling sore. The thought of new tricks wasn't so appealing at the moment!

But I said, "Yeah, maybe."

I sat down and stretched my hamstrings, mainly watching other people do various exercises with the small weighted balls. It looked a little more fun than my old weight routine.

I used to read some of the men's fitness magazines, so I used to at least have an idea of new trends in working out. But some of this was new to me.

"Ready to go?" Jim asked.

"Yes. If I want to walk home on my own power, I'd better stop now," I joked.

With a wave to Megan on the way out and a couple of brochures in hand, we were on our way home.

"So how was that?" Jim asked.

"Great. Yeah," I replied, upbeat. "Thanks for taking me. I'll have to look into a membership for us."

"You hated it," he said knowingly.

"Yeah."

CHAPTER 31

Okay okay, I didn't hate going to the gym. Jim had been joking (sort of).

But I didn't love it.

Years ago, back when I had a little more time, I used to drag myself to the gym with my friends, and it was okay, because we were all there.

I could make myself go, bring some music to work out with, have workout buddies, and all that.

But while some of my friends could live at the gym, to me it was a grind.

And this time I wanted to be smarter about working out. I didn't want another gym membership that was going to gather dust.

As we walked and ran (mainly walked) home, we got talking about working out and keeping fit, and why it was so tough to stick with it.

"You've got to really pick something that you like," Jim said, stating the obvious.

"I used to like going to the gym, enough to make myself go," I countered. "I think it's just a matter of getting back into a routine with it."

"What did you like about it?"

"Uh, I um" I stumbled over my words. (I was usually a little more eloquent!)

He eased to a stop in front of our houses.

"Well, I used to like going with friends," I started. "It felt good after I was done, like an accomplishment. I got pretty strong for playing hoops."

"Yeah, it's too bad that you couldn't enjoy the activity itself, not just the feeling of being done. But you know that resilient people do focus on the outcome and that keeps them going. So, besides finding something you enjoy, this is a good strategy to keep in mind," Jim commented.

Hmm. Good point.

"Some of the stuff you were doing looked pretty cool," I told him, stretching my shoulders. (They already felt sore!)

"It's amazing, and way more interesting than what I used to do" Jim said. "The personal trainer I worked with is excellent. He jokingly told me that I graduated, but I check in with him once in a while, just to shake it up. I can give you his contact info."

"That would be great," I said, trying to sound enthused.

"He might also be able to help you find some other activities that you would really enjoy," Jim added.

"Dad!" Our front door opened, and David ran out, basketball in hand, to me.

"Hi Jim," he pumped energetically.

"Hey David," Jim said warmly. "Are you having a great day?"

"Yep!"

David dropped the basketball as I picked him up, groaning jokingly. "Did you grow overnight?"

"I just had some yogurt with blueberries," he explained seriously.

"That's got to be it," Jim winked. He reached over and squeezed David's bicep while David flexed proudly. David's arms look like they belong on a Muppet, which made it extra cute.

"Want to play basketball with me, Dad?"

"Sure, sounds fun." And it did.

I put him down and he picked up the basketball again, dribbling it a few times.

I loved that David had discovered basketball. It certainly helped to have Ty and Kim and their kids around to play with.

"Ty told me that your dad is a pretty good basketball player," Jim said to David.

"Yeah he's pretty good," David said, tugging me a little toward the house. The basketball looked huge tucked under his arm.

I chuckled. "I think Ty was being kind in his comments," I said to Jim. "He's amazing. So is Kim for that matter!"

"Yes, they're fantastic athletes. So cool that they still love to play."

"You can see how much they love it when they're goofing around with the kids," I agreed.

David leaned against me and sighed.

Jim ruffled his hair and patted me on the back. "Thanks for coming with me," he said.

"Thanks so much Jim. I appreciate it," I told him sincerely, as he crossed the street. I grabbed the basketball from David, dribbled it a couple of times, then did a little bounce pass to him.

"Sounds like one of your favorite activities is right under your nose," Jim called behind his back.

CHAPTER 32

A little while later, David and I were at the park, shooting hoops and goofing around.

There are a few basketball hoops there, some set a little lower for kids.

A few of the neighborhood teenagers were there, and a few other parents and kids. There was a nice atmosphere.

"What did Jim mean when he said one of your favorite activities is under your nose?" David asked, dribbling erratically around me. "Did he mean me?"

"Yeah, I think he meant playing with you," I agreed, winking. "And it's really cool that you like to play basketball, because that was my favorite sport as a kid."

"Why isn't it now?"

David passed me the ball with the question.

I dribbled the ball from one hand to the other between my legs, then showed David a simple way to do it with little legs.

"I guess it still is," I said thoughtfully.

"Why don't you play anymore?"

I bounce passed the ball to him. "Boing," I said as it bounced. We passed it back and forth with a few 'boings' as it bounced.

Then he went in for a jump shot, hitting the rim with the ball and covering his head with his arms as it ricocheted back down.

"Ahh," he half-yelled.

"It's okay," I told him. "Just keep your hands up and keep watching the ball. Then you can get the rebound."

"Okay," he said gamely, dribbling to the net again. He shot another one, and I caught the rebound, passing it back to David.

"So why don't you play?" he asked again.

"There hasn't been a lot of time, buddy," I told him.

"So play with me," he said seriously.

I smiled. "I always have time to play with you."

And these days, I thought proudly, I did.

As we walked off the court, one of the moms approached me. "You must coach basketball," she commented.

"Not really," I laughed. "Just this guy."

"My dad is super good at basketball," David chimed in.

I laughed again. "I've taught him well," I joked.

"You've got a really good approach," she said. "I'm Jenny by the way. We live just over here. You all just moved in a few months ago?"

I nodded. "We love the neighborhood. I'm Alex, and this is David. My wife's name is Joan. Joanie."

"Nice to meet you both. Yes, you moved in across from Jim and Vanessa?"

"Yes," I said enthusiastically.

"Aren't they amazing," she said, in a statement, not a question.

"That's an understatement," I laughed, and Jenny did too. "I can tell that everyone loves them."

Just then, Joanie came strolling towards us. "Hey guys," she called out as she approached.

I put my hand on her shoulder affectionately and introduced her to Jenny.

"I noticed how much fun these two were having," Jenny told Joanie. "There's a really great junior basketball club here, if you ever want to get involved. Playing or coaching."

"I'm too young to coach," David told her, straight-faced, even though I think he was joking.

"You're adorable," Jenny said directly to David. Then to me, "If you're ever interested, my husband's involved. He can give you some info."

We all chatted for a moment, until the ultimate conversation ender came from David.

"I've got to go to the bathroom."

CHAPTER 33

That night at dinner, we talked about the day as we ate grilled vegetables and salmon with a mango salsa.

Joanie used to do pilates and dance. She had started going to pilates again, and had gone to a great class at a new studio that Kim had recommended.

She used to dance around the kitchen when we'd cook. (She's actually got great rhythm. I just kind of shuffle and clap like an orangutan.)

That afternoon, when David and I came into the kitchen after putting his swing up, it was really cool to see her dancing around again, dance music blasting.

"Wow, Mom's funny," David commented to me, laughing.

"What? I'm awesome," Joanie had said, picking him up and dancing with him.

"Just agree buddy," I had joked, as she tried to get me to dance. It was fun to just goof around.

Joanie was more relaxed and upbeat in general, the way she was when we were dating and first married.

I don't know how much of that was the lifestyle changes we had made, and how much was her new outlook with wanting to quit her job and find work that meant something to her. Whatever the combination, it was awesome to see her happy, relaxed, and optimistic – her usual dynamic self.

We went outside after dinner, and checked our garden. It looked lush and healthy. David pointed out every new cucumber and pea pod to us.

Then Joanie and I sat on the patio while David counted our tomatoes. (He was becoming a serious gardener!)

Our conversation turned to the day's activities.

"You know, I think David is really going to get into basketball," I told Joanie. "He picks up the skills so easily."

"You said I was awesome, Dad," David called from the garden.

Someone was getting big ears.

"You are awesome buddy," I called back.

Joanie smiled. "He told me how much he loved playing with you," she agreed. "You should take him out more often."

"Yeah you should, Dad," David cut in.

"I was thinking afterward, all afternoon in fact, how much fun it was to teach him some skills," I said quietly to Joanie. "Remember when I told you I used to volunteer at the Y in high school? I loved teaching basketball there, and working with the kids."

"You should get involved then," she coaxed. "Ty and Kim must know some good clubs for kids."

"Yeah," I nodded. "And that neighbor, Jenny, said her husband coaches with a group. As long as it's fun for David. I mean, I haven't coached for years," I trailed off.

"You don't have to be an NBA coach. You're keen and good with kids. You were a really good high school player, and you've worked with kids before," Joanie said. Then, rubbing my shoulder, she said sweetly, "You're the whole package, baby."

Reowr.

"What are you saying? I can't hear you?"

Yes, our little eavesdropper.

"Hey, you want to come up here and join the conversation?" Joanie asked.

"No," David said innocently. But he came up, climbed up on Joanie's lap and snuggled in.

"Maybe we'll start some basketball in the fall, David," I suggested. "Like, a skills and drills group or something like that."

"You and me?"

"Well, you," I corrected. "Because you want to play with other kids your age."

"Yeah, I want to do that," David nodded. "And you should coach us."

"Yeah? Well I just might," I smiled. "But it would also be fun for you to have other coaches too. That way you won't get too sick of me."

I winked at Joanie as David nodded.

We sat for a moment. But kids can never sit still for long.

"I'm bored," David said.

Usually after supper, we'd watch a movie or some t.v. but Joanie had started trying to break out of doing that every night.

"How about we play a game," she offered.

"Can we play The Game of Life?" David asked.

"Oh yeah, we just picked that up this week," Joanie told me. "Yes, that sounds fun."

"I'm in," I added.

I remembered playing The Game of Life when I was younger. Your game pieces are various color cars, and you 'drive' along the board with your pink or blue stick figure in your car (yeah, I know: gender stereotyping at its best), rolling the dice to see what you'll land on: marriage, kids, a new job, a bigger house.

A little while later, we were all cruising around the game board. We had all chosen our jobs: I was a carpenter, David was an actor (because you can pretend and get money for it, as he informed us) and Joan was a teacher.

"Why aren't you a teacher in real life, Mom?"

"Well, I had an interest in business, so I went to business school," she answered.

"But don't you just walk around all day and carry a laptop?" he followed.

Joanie and I laughed. Some days I felt like that, and obviously she did too.

"Maybe I might want to teach people how to do business," Joanie thought out loud.

"Fun," David said.

Joanie smiled, and I could tell the wheels were turning. I looked at her, and made a mental note to chat with her about that later. I was happy that she was moving forward.

As David rolled on 'twins', he exclaimed, "Oh yeah, more kids!"

He was driving a full car.

"We should have more kids," David told us. He looked back and forth between us. "What do you think?"

"Uhhh," Joanie and I both said at the same time.

Truth is, a few months ago, the thought of another kid was non-existent. Joanie and I had been so busy, stressed, and tuned out from each other. But these days, I wondered…

As we stuttered through the beginning of a response, David moved on, focusing again on the game, and his little stick figures.

"I'll name you "Tree" and you "Leaf", he announced.

Joanie and I grinned at each other. Hmm, hopefully his naming skills would improve before he had real kids.

"Awesome buddy," Joanie said.

David was moving his car around. "Come on Sunshine," he said. "Let's go to the beach."

"Who's," I started.

"My wife, Dad," David said seriously. "Her name is Sunshine."

"Cool," I nodded.

"Yeah, and I think I win," David continued, still moving his car all over the place, "because I have a really happy family and we're going to go get ice cream and do fun things together, and you're going to come over and stay with us! And we'll play basketball a lot."

David sat back, pretty pleased with himself.

Those sweet thoughts from our five year old had some wisdom.

The more balance I attained, the more I put into relationships, the healthier my habits became, the happier I was.

I felt like I was starting to win at the real game of life.

CHAPTER 34

A few weeks went by, and, although we had some hiccups, in general my life and our life together was moving in a more positive direction.

As Jim kept telling me, real change doesn't necessarily happen overnight. It's a process, complete with speed bumps, and sometimes, even a barrier.

"Lots of ways to get past an obstacle," Jim would say. "Why do you think people climb fences?"

My weekly lunches with Jim were something I looked forward to, and not just because he was giving me such valuable life advice.

Sometimes we just chatted about this and that. Jim had become a close friend as well as a mentor.

I never thought I'd say that about a guy a few decades older than me, but Jim was kind of ageless. In fact, since he was volunteering with some teenagers at the YMCA, he actually sounded way younger than me sometimes.

Case in point: We were having lunch last week, and I told Jim that David was starting skills and drills in September. I had spoken with Kim and Ty and a few others, and I was going to start coaching basketball in the same junior league.

"As the kids at the Y say, that's really lit, Alex," he declared.

"Is that a good thing?" I asked, chuckling.

"Oh yeah, it's the best," Jim affirmed, shrugging.

"I've obviously got to get cooler to hang out with you, Jim," I laughed. (I was semi-serious!)

"You're going in the right direction, Alex," Jim said. "Kids always keep you on your toes. You're going to feel great."

I nodded, agreeing.

I was already feeling great. Summer was winding down, but the fall was going to be all about new beginnings.

David was excited about starting school, and had met his teacher. He had also met a few of the neighborhood kids his age, so he'd have some pals, and meet some new friends too.

Joanie was quietly putting out her feelers, meeting with various old friends and mentors. She had connected with a few new people, and had quite a few individuals tell her to get in touch when she was ready to make a move. She was holding her cards close to her chest though. She wanted a positive, flexible work situation.

We had decided not to take a big, expensive vacation this year. We ended up renting a little cottage at the beach for a few days. Kim and Ty came out with the kids for an overnight, and my sister and her family rented a place nearby.

Six months ago, the thought of going to the beach with my sister would have given me a headache.

Once I didn't care about 'keeping up with the Joneses', it was just fun to re-connect. I think they appreciated how low key and relaxed the vacation was.

I had forgotten how sweet Em's kids are, and what a nice guy Glen is.

And I had forgotten how much fun Emily is.

One day when we were digging clams on the beach with the kids, she thanked me for suggesting the getaway.

"Why haven't we done this before?" Emily asked.

"I think I've been too caught up with work," I told her. "And stuff."

"Yeah, me too," she said. "I feel like I have to keep up with everything all the time. Our house, lessons for the kids, work…"

"According to Mom, your life is perfect," I told Em, laughing.

Emily rolled eyes. "Don't get me wrong," she said. "I love Mom, but she's about to drive me crazy. Glen and I had a big talk after their last visit. He told me I shouldn't have to try so hard with my own mother. And I agree. I'm trying to make my life more simple, and the kids' lives more simple. Play more, hang out more, don't worry about unimportant stuff."

"Wow."

"Can you tell I have a life coach?" she grinned.

"That's good!"

"It actually is good," she nodded.

"I get it, Em. It gets exhausting, trying to keep up," I agreed. "And it just moves you away from what makes you really happy and what you value."

I told her about Jim, and what a good influence he'd been.

We paused, that comfortable silence as we dug in the sand.

"I missed you," she told me.

"Me too," I said sincerely.

"You missed yourself?" she goofed around, grinning.

"No, you, dummy," I shot back.

That got me a clump of sand on the head.

Thirty seconds later, I'm chasing her around the beach as the kids shriek with laughter. (I also forgot how fast she is!)

The best parts of the holiday were all the simple things: campfires in the evenings, hanging out on the beach, jumping around in the waves, watching our kids play.

CHAPTER 35

By the end of the summer, I was feeling pretty optimistic. I really noticed the change on Mondays. For one thing, I was waking up without that familiar stab in my chest – stress at the impending week.

Maybe that was because I was sleeping though the night these days. No more waking up at three in the morning, wheels turning with a million little worries.

This particular Monday, I was walking towards my building when my phone beeped with a text. It was from Sam, my old business school buddy.

After running into Sam and Bridgette at the market a few weeks back, we wanted to make sure we re-connected. So we had gotten together a few times. Just yesterday, we organized a hike and potluck lunch with them and their kids.

We had all brought trail food to share, met at a park, hiked in to a picnic area on some trails, and had lunch and chatted while the kids played. Their kids were a lot of fun - just like Sam and Bridgette.

Thx for ystrdy! You all free on 18th? Our place.

As I was replying, I got another text, this one from Jim.

I had texted him yesterday to say thanks again. Jim had, as promised, given me the contact info for that personal trainer.

You're welcome! How's it going?

The trainer's name was Phil and we had already met twice. Phil was pretty busy, so it had taken a few weeks to get an appointment, but Jim had put in a good word.

The first time, we just chatted. He wanted to know all about my background, and just get familiar with each other.

I used to think of personal trainers as just big guys or gals that pushed you in the gym or coached you. But Phil and I talked about past experiences, lifestyle, and my goals. We chatted about Joanie and David, and about work.

By the end of the conversation, I felt really positive about moving forward.

Phil really knew his stuff, and had more letters behind his name than I did, plus a degree in exercise science. I was in.

The second time we met up, we actually did go to the gym (at my request) and did some general conditioning and worked with weighted balls and bosu balls, etc. He showed me all these exercises that I could do anywhere.

Phil and I also talked about general physical activity, and making my day more active. I was already going in the right direction, with active lunches, taking the stairs, and that sort of thing. I thought Bryan was going to flip his lid (or at least mock me continuously) when I brought an exercise ball into my office to sit on. But it was another little change. (Try sitting on a large exercise ball at your desk, and tell me it doesn't make you use your muscles more and have better posture!)

According to Phil, it didn't have to be a scheduled workout or trip to the gym every time.

Saying that, Joanie and I had signed up for tennis lessons at the community courts.

I was really looking forward to connecting with Phil again, later this week.

I had that great nervous anticipation, like I used to get when I was trying out for a basketball team.

Speaking of basketball, I felt a new sense of excitement about David's burgeoning love of playing. I didn't want to be that dad who shoved his favorite sport down his kid's throat. As long as he was having fun.

I stopped for a moment to reply to Jim. Then I looked up. It was a sunny day with no wind. Just perfect.

The downtown business association had planted trees a few years ago, trying to make the area more attractive. It had worked. There were lots of trees, grassy areas, and benches.

I was trying to be more mindful of my surroundings these days. Stop and smell the roses, as they say. Or, in this case, feel the sun on my face, and listen to the birds in the trees for a moment.

One of the guys on my floor came striding out of our building. He hadn't been at the company for long, but seemed to be pretty pleasant and a hard worker.

I snapped out of it, thinking I should get in there and start on a few emails. I was trying to be pro-active and feel more in control, as opposed to arriving at work feeling panicked, like I used to.

I waved at the guy as he saw me and diverted toward me.

"Hey," I started. Think, what was his name?

"Jack," I finished. (Yes! Score one for a clear noggin!)

Jack's eyes were a little wide and he looked a little freaked out. That reminded me of a certain someone a few months ago. (Yes, me!)

"Did you hear anything, Alex?" he asked as he got within speaking distance.

"About what?" I asked.

He really looked stressed.

"They're meeting with the heads of each pod this morning. Word just came down from head office about possible cuts."

"What? That's probably just a rumor," I said calmly, as I pulled out my phone and hit the email icon.

There it was: an email from my boss to Bryan, me, and a couple of the other guys who were group leaders. The head honchos had met to discuss 'cost-saving measures'.

Then a text from Bryan:

Where r u? Doodoo hitting fan

I got that stab in my chest that I hadn't been missing.

"This is going to be bad," Jack said ominously. I realized he was still standing there.

I took a deep breath. "Let's just see," I started, then trailed off.

Jack shook his head. "I'm going to get doughnuts," he informed me. "We're going to need something to cheer everyone up."

Here we go again, I thought cynically. I looked at my watch. It was eight-thirty in the morning, and that old feeling of defeat had just returned.

CHAPTER 36

I took the elevator, partly because of the irrational fear that the stabbing pain in my chest was a heart attack.

Mainly, the elevator was there and I just wanted to get upstairs and see what was going on.

As I walked onto the floor, everyone looked upset, or at least a little extra tense.

I saw Bryan and Will talking in Bryan's office doorway, and high-tailed it over.

"What's going on?" I asked.

Bryan looked grim and Will looked nervous. Bryan wasn't our boss per se, but he was the senior executive in our area. He definitely had the scoop.

"Come on in," Bryan instructed both of us as we sat down.

"There are going to be cuts today," Bryan told us. You two are, from what I've heard, safe."

Will breathed a sigh of relief. Bryan sat behind his desk and leaned back, running his hands through his greying hair. It was probably going to get greyer after today.

"Alex, as a group leader, you're protected," Bryan continued. "Will, you've accumulated just enough seniority to be okay. Plus, your performance has been excellent." Bryan looked at me after he said that to Will, as if my performance was somehow lacking. Strangely it was up across the board, but funny how old-school perception still exists because I'm not there at all hours anymore.

"So who's getting cut?" I asked. I leaned back in my chair. Maybe this wouldn't be so bad. Big companies shuffled things around every so often.

"They're cutting a dozen people, mainly junior employees and a couple of trainees, but I heard that Jessica is gone."

"Jessica," Will repeated. "She's brilliant!"

"Too many 'working from home' days, and the stress was getting to her. She had too much going on outside of work and it interfered."

"What? That's crazy," I complained.

"They've been looking at performance and cost ratios, and they're not happy," Bryan said seriously. "There's a lot of competition out there, and we used to be the leaders. Now we're middle of the pack."

Bryan looked directly at me again.

"We're going to have to put on our big boy pants and step it up, particularly you, Alex, as a group leader," he advised. "We'll all have to shoulder an extra workload, but you also need to let people see your face around here. A lot."

Truth is, I wasn't the first in and the last out everyday anymore, but I was incredibly focused and effective when I was at work. My pod was working well together. We had even started doing one meeting a day outside. Something about getting out of the office, the fresh air, the movement —

something – that had made them happier and more productive.

Anyway, point taken.

We all got up.

I felt like I had a cloud over my head.

Just when I'm working my ass off to get some balance in my life, and just when I'm starting to feel better, work takes a big bite out of all my efforts.

An hour ago, I had control over my life again. Now, all I felt was a crushing weight on my shoulders.

I couldn't win.

CHAPTER 37

I'd like to say the rest of the day flew by, but it didn't. It crawled.

I went into my office and sat down at my desk. I could feel myself slouching in my seat the way I used to do.

I had forgotten how crappy it was to feel powerless, depressed, and stressed – all at the same time.

"Get it together," I told myself.

I sat up straight and took a deep breath. Then I texted my pod to meet in ten minutes.

Where were my Tums?

I opened my drawer and rooted around, finding an almost full bottle. Now, I sensed, they wouldn't last for long.

I popped a couple in my mouth, and glanced at the picture of Joan, David, and me on my desk. It was a new one that Joan gave me, in a sleek silver frame. We had been hiking.

Then I looked at it again. We were all grinning like fools. I remember how I felt that day: just so free and happy. It was the simplest of days, sunny and warm. Easy conversation with friends as we walked.

I looked away. When were those Tums going to kick in?

I organized some of my papers and did a mental checklist of what I wanted to discuss with my group.

Then I sat back and tuned in to how I was feeling.

I know I know, that sounds kind of 'new age'.

It was something my trainer, Phil, had recommended. He had actually recommended meditation, but I had joked that I'd get laughed out of my office (by Bryan) if I started sitting on some mat and meditating.

So he had suggested starting by taking five minutes each day, closing my office door, and just tuning out everything else. With me, it was difficult, so I concentrated on my breathing. 5 seconds in and 5 seconds out, feeling the air move in and out.

For doing something seemingly so small, it had already started to make an amazing difference.

Right now though, I was breathing fast and shallow.

It always took me a minute or two to quiet my mind enough to slow myself down. Today, there were too many scenarios running through it – most of them involving me stuck at this f'ing desk.

There was a knock.

So much for five minutes.

"Come in," I barked, not meaning to.

The door opened and my three junior advisors tumbled into my office. They all had that shitty wide-eyed look of stress that I've had so many times before.

"Everyone grab a seat," I told them grimly.

I outlined our plan for the foreseeable future. More cuts could be coming. We were going to have to outperform the other pods if we wanted to have some stability.

They nodded like sad puppies and it made me feel all the more depressed.

"Everything's going to be okay," I finished.

The problem was, I didn't just want 'okay' anymore.

CHAPTER 38

After my meeting, I walked over to check in with Jessica, and wish her well.

Inside I was slouching, but I tried to walk tall and convey an attitude that it was business as usual.

Bryan strode up. "Hey, one of the interns is doing a burger run," he said quickly. "You want a special?"

A special wasn't feeling so special anymore. Since I had gotten away from the old double burger, fries, and soft drink, I hadn't missed them.

Until now.

I used to operate pretty well on what I called 'stress food'.

"I don't think they have any celery salads there," Bryan joked, mocking my recent healthy eating.

"Yeah, just grab me a special, thanks," I shot back, trying to sound appreciative that he had asked.

I got to Jessica's office. She was wrapping her framed pictures in paper. It looked like she had most of her other personal items boxed up.

She looked strangely calm.

I poked my head in the doorway.

"Hey, Jessica," I started, not sure how to follow.

"Hey Alex," she said crisply.

"I'm sorry to hear," I started again, and trailed off.

"I'm not," Jessica stated, looking directly at me.

I wasn't sure how to respond.

"This place is freaking toxic at times," she continued.

She pointed to the remaining pictures on her desk. "You know why I'm wrapping these up last," she asked. "To remind myself how much I sacrificed for this company. Every time I start to feel bad, I look at the picture of my family. Oh yeah, even my dog will get to know me again now."

"Yeah, exactly," I soothed. "And it's good to vent."

"Oh I'm not venting," she shot back. "I'm stating the truth. I cannot believe I stayed here so long. This company almost sucked the life right out of me. This is my new opportunity. I want to do it differently."

I smiled wistfully. I actually felt a tinge of jealousy. "You've been amazing to work with, Jess. You've taught me a lot."

"I was really starting to like our walking meetings," she said, smiling at me.

"The higher ups just don't get it yet, do they," I said. "That we don't have to be chained to a desk all day to be productive."

She shook her head. "Nope."

I stepped forward and hugged her. "Take care and keep in touch."

She nodded. "Say hi to Joanie, will you? And give that little scrumptious David a hug when you get home tonight."

I nodded and started to go.

"Alex," she called.

I turned around.

"Don't let it happen to you again."

"Don't let what happen?"

She looked at me square in the eye. "Don't let work become your life again. I've seen a tremendous change in you over the past few months. Don't let anyone take that away from you."

I nodded, unsettled by how happy Jessica was to get out of here.

CHAPTER 39

I had texted Joanie about the shake up at work, and that I'd be home late. Still, I was hoping to say goodnight to David before he went to sleep.

When I pulled in the driveway, I had a real sense of déjà vu. So I wasn't surprised when I walked in, and Joanie met me, with her finger to her lips in that universal quiet signal – David had just fallen asleep.

Yes, I had been here many times. And it felt pretty bad.

She kissed me. "What happened?" she asked softly, as I took off my jacket.

"There were cuts at work," I explained, trying to keep my voice calm. "The rest of us have to step it up."

I walked straight to the cupboard and took down a can of Coke. We didn't buy many soft drinks anymore, just for when we had company. I got the bottle of rum also, and two glasses.

"Want one?" I asked.

"Sure," she said gamely.

She got some ice cubes and lemon, and I made the drinks.

"Want some supper?" she asked sweetly. I could tell she was treading lightly around me, which made me feel worse.

"We all got burgers at work," I said, rubbing my chest.

"Want to sit on the deck?" Joanie asked.

I sighed. "No, not really."

Honestly, I felt so shitty, all I could do was wallow in it. Going out on the deck now would just remind me that I wasn't going to see much leisure time for a while. I know that sounds childish, but it would just make me feel worse.

We went into the family room and sat on the couch. We talked about the uncertainty at work and the increased workload. A couple of months ago, I would have kept it all in, but it felt better to talk to Joan about it. I also wanted her to know how bad this development made me feel. Things had been going so well.

Joanie had her legs curled under her, facing me. She put her hand on the back of my neck and rubbed it for a minute. I closed my eyes for a few seconds.

"Jessica's gone," I said.

"What? Really?"

"She was happy about it, too," I followed. "At first I thought she was just really pissed off, but I think she was just charged up."

"Wow," she said, shaking her head. "She's so amazing. Smart, savvy, positive. The whole package."

Joanie looked a little shaken. She was probably thinking the same thing I was: If Jessica was dispensable, so was I.

"She said to say hi to you by the way," I added. "Asked how you were doing."

Joan nodded, distracted.

"I was going to have coffee with her soon," Joanie said, half to herself. "But that's probably not a good idea now." She trailed off.

"She'll have a lot more time to have coffee now," I shot back sarcastically.

Joan shifted on the couch. "No, I mean, since I was looking at other options for work," Joan reminded me. "You know how I was going to think about working part time?"

I took a deep breath.

"But I'll put that on hold for a while," she added.

I looked at her, feeling guilty. "Maybe that's a good idea. I just can't handle any more uncertainty right now. At least your job is stable."

Joan nodded but her face sunk just a little.

"Everything's going to be okay," she soothed.

She got up. "Why don't you come to bed and get a good night's sleep. Things will settle in again."

"You go ahead," I told her.

She kissed me, and went to bed while I sat there.

Then I got myself another drink.

CHAPTER 40

I cancelled lunch with Jim on Tuesday.

For the rest of the week, I felt like an old man. I didn't work out, I ate like crap, and I worked a bunch of extra hours, although I didn't feel like I got more done. In fact, I had been more productive before the cuts.

Everyone in my office looked awful too. No one was really talking about the cuts. We all just had our heads down.

By the time Bryan, Will, and I met some of the other guys in the office for lunch on Friday, I was effectively back to square one.

(No, I actually felt worse these days, because I had put so much effort into feeling better and living better, and just gotten a taste of how good things could be… Only to have it snatched away.)

I said a mental 'screw it' as I ordered a double bacon cheeseburger, and listened to Bryan drone on about how lucky we all were.

On the way back to the office, Will and I walked together. Will's usually a pretty chipper guy, but I could tell something was on his mind.

"Hey, I hope you're not letting the cuts bother you," I said quietly. "You're doing a great job. We just have to ride it out."

I was about to go on, when he looked me square in the eye. We slowed down, and a couple of the guys passed us.

"Ashley's pregnant," he said, in a low voice.

"That's fantastic," I pumped, patting him on the back. This was something they had wanted for a long time.

He didn't answer right away.

"You must be excited," I said.

(Will did not look excited.)

"I am, but things at work have really rattled me," he told me. "Ash is planning to stop working once the baby comes, but I'm worried that if things aren't stable at work, she won't be able to," he went on.

"You're doing a great job," I told him. "The worst is over."

"The other thing is, I want to actually be around for the baby. Not working like crazy," he admitted. "I don't want to be the absent father."

Bryan strode past us. "Let's go boys," he boomed, teasing. "Don't go getting slack already!"

I didn't feel like laughing. By the look on Will's face, neither did he.

CHAPTER 41

The next week was still dismal at work, and it wasn't doing a lot for my state of mind.

I canceled lunch again with Jim, telling him that things were crazy at work, and I couldn't slack off.

"You know, eating's not slacking off, Alex," Jim had kidded gently. "Neither is getting some exercise."

"I know," I had started. I didn't finish.

"Let me know if you want to chat," he told me. "Anytime."

The drag was, I wanted to be able to talk with Jim more now than before. How had he navigated through this crap when he was working?

My mind was all over the place. I was pissed off, tired, nervous, defeated. I wanted to throw my phone against a wall. And, as funny as this sounds, I was actually lonely.

Some people can work well under pressure, and maybe I'm one of them, but I hated it. I wasn't a lot of fun to be around.

You know how people say we behave at our worst around the people we love most?

Well, that was me.

I was short with Joanie, grumpy around the house, and, although I was trying to be present with David, I kept saying stuff like, "Daddy's got a lot on his mind right now," to which David would respond with a quizzical look.

Then he'd go find Joan.

It was like work stress, long hours, and guilt (at not being able to spend more quality time with David and Joanie, and Joan not feeling like she could leave her job now) was knocking all the energy out of me. I fell asleep in front of the TV more times than I care to admit.

Joanie and David were trying to be understanding, but I'm sure they weren't surprised at the fact that I was back to my old habits.

I had tried to change a few times before, but this time I really thought it would be different.

It wasn't.

I had failed. I felt helpless again.

Or at least that was what I thought, until I had that late night conversation with – you guessed it – Jim.

It was Friday night, around eleven. I was sitting on the front step, effectively feeling sorry for myself.

I had scrambled to make it home to read to David before bed, but I fell asleep pretty quickly. When I woke up, the lights were all off and Joanie had gone to bed.

She had gotten past being sympathetic, then angry at me for not being around. Now, again, she just didn't expect me to be around. She actually said I was throwing off their routine when I showed up.

Anyway, so there I was, sitting there, sipping on a cold one, trying to clear my head enough to go to bed and actually sleep, when I heard a door open across the street.

A dark bundle of fur came scrambling out of Jim and Vanessa's door, followed by Jim.

"Forest," he called softly, and the bundle of fur came back to him. Jim put him on a leash.

I sat up straighter. "Hey. Jim," I called. When he looked over, I waved. He waved back.

"Come on Forest," he coaxed, as they started toward me. Forest looked like a golden retriever. He was a beautiful dog.

"Hey Alex," Jim said softly. (The windows were open.) "This is Forest."

Forest was looking pretty perky for almost midnight. I gave him a pat and an ear rub.

"Hi Forest," I said softly. Then to Jim, "Where'd you get this handsome guy?"

"Gal," Jim corrected me.

I chuckled. "She's beautiful."

"She is, isn't she," Jim smiled. "She's my daughter's baby. They're on vacation, so Forest gets to stay with Gramma and Grampa." (He said the last part to Forest, in a voice you'd use for a baby.) Forest wagged her tail like crazy in response.

He patted her head. "She's always a little extra excited on the first night with us."

I nodded and patted her again. She liked me. "David's been after us for a dog," I told Jim.

"Send him over tomorrow," Jim said. "He can play with her and help take care of her if he wants to."

"Thanks, he'd love that." I smiled into a sigh.

Jim looked at me. "I saw you sitting out here. How are you?"

I sighed out an "Oh," then said, "I've been better."

I told him about the cuts at work, the new workload, and the uncertainty.

He nodded knowingly. "I figured. I've been there," he said simply.

"I'd offer you a beer or some water, but I'm not sure Forest wants to hang out," I added.

"Want to come for a walk with us?" Jim asked.

Forest looked game.

Stretching my legs, I nodded. "Let me just lock the door and grab a key."

We walked for an hour.

The first part was me griping about the frustration of trying to live well, and (in my mind) failing; of not being in control of my life, and of seeing my coping skills drop.

Jim nodded. He nodded a lot. But he didn't say anything.

In a weird way, I felt a little smug: I had stumped him. Not everyone could live the way Jim talked about.

"I've tried," I finished venting. "But some things are out of your control."

Jim nodded again, and smiled.

Then he started talking.

"There's something that I've seen in you, and you need to remember it," he said. "It's resilience."

I was listening.

"Everyone is going to have tough times or setbacks. That's a given. If you're a resilient person, you're going to bounce back."

"I think I've lost my elasticity, Jim," I half-joked, half-whined.

"Two things that resilient people have are: They have the ability to problem solve, and they have optimism," Jim told me. "You have both of those, Alex. You're a smart guy. You're a positive guy. You take those characteristics, and use them as tools to help you bounce back."

I didn't say anything. I was processing it.

"Sometimes you have to work at being resilient," Jim continued. "It's a process, like exercising to get fitter. But there are strategies you can use, like a mental toolbox."

"Like what?" I asked. I had started the walk in a pretty low mood, but now I was intrigued.

"For instance, you can do an exercise called: 'on the plate, off the plate', by yourself or with Joanie," Jim said. "You can only fit so much on your plate, right?"

"Right," I nodded.

"This is basically prioritizing," Jim explained. "You have to start by assessing what's important to you."

I nodded again.

"It sounds like you've talked to Joanie about what you both want in the big picture."

I nodded.

"As long as you have that vision and know what you value," Jim continued, "you just keep going in that direction. There will always be roadblocks. Just detour around them and get back on track."

"Or push through," I said, grinning.

"That's the spirit, Alex," Jim encouraged. He chuckled. "Just don't go through any roadblocks for real. I'll tell you about the colleague of mine, and his BMW 7 series, sometime. He needed to talk to someone, before he took that baby for a ride."

Forest wagged her tail, reacting to his tone. He bent down and scratched behind her ear.

At the end of our walk, we were standing on the side of the street, between our houses. I patted Forest. After I had thanked him for yet more wisdom, he left me with one last thing.

"You're not powerless, Alex."

Then he and Forest went in, the retriever wagging her tail as if she agreed.

CHAPTER 42

The next morning, Saturday, I was tired. But I got up pretty early and found David reading in his bed. We started breakfast together.

When Joanie got up, I gave her a big hug, which surprised her and made David giggle. "I'm sorry I've let things slip," I said softly to her. "Let's take some time today and talk."

"You're not working?" she asked, teeth still a little clenched. (This was going to take a little time!)

"Nope, not today. Then to both of them, "Let's go to the farmer's market."

David was pumped. "Yeah!"

"Your mother called last night," Joanie said, her jaw still set. "They're coming in overnight."

"Oh," I responded.

She grabbed a banana and started to peel it fairly ferociously. She dumped it in our blender. I looked at David, and he shrugged and gave me this cartoonish wide-eyed look, as if to say, 'I don't know why she's mad at you'.

"Don't we have plans?" I asked.

"We did, with Kim and Ty and the kids, but I didn't even know if you'd want to keep them anyway," Joanie said tersely.

'On the plate, off the plate', I thought.

"I'll call my folks," I told Joan.

And I did. I told them they were welcome to come and stay with us, but we had already made plans. They could watch a movie and relax.

When my dad said he had to take Mom to the mall, so we could grab a burger and beer while she shopped, I politely declined. I was taking David to play basketball.

Joanie, David and I went to the market that morning. And we had a great time. We bought healthy food. He danced to a local guy playing the fiddle. And we saw some friends.

Later, while David played in the yard with a couple of pals, Joanie and I had a good talk and revisited what we really wanted.

We both agreed it wasn't having the biggest house or the fanciest car, or any of that.

So we decided not to wait for her to resign from her job.

Then my folks arrived, and Mom started going on about my brother-in-law's new Porsche SUV. I was happy for Glen. (And, don't get me wrong, I wouldn't turn down a Porsche SUV, but I realized it was getting lower on my priority list.)

Then I invited my parents to come to the playground with David and I. We played basketball, and Mom and Dad cheered David on. We had a nice walk.

That night, we ordered them a pizza and went over to Kim and Ty's with David.

And we had a nice weekend.

On Monday, Joanie quit her job and met with Jessica. She came home excited about starting to do some consulting and that they might start a business together. She had a spark of excitement that I hadn't seen for a while.

I didn't cancel lunch with Jim on Tuesday.

I had an efficient morning at the office, then had a really invigorating lunch and walk with him.

I was telling him about how my mother, in our last conversation, had told me I should quit my job if it was stressing me out so much, and start a new one. Jim laughed as I recounted our back and forth.

Then he said something so perceptive:

"You don't want to quit your job, Alex."

I was surprised at his candor.

"Well, besides the fact that I've already put in years at this position, and I'm on track for a VP position in the future," I started.

"Yeah, for sure," he interrupted politely. "But you've worked hard, and you value your work there, and you're excellent at it. I can tell from our conversations. Plus I hear things," he added, grinning.

"Well, yeah," I stuttered. "But I'd kind of feel bad saying that I value work over other stuff."

"But you can value your work. You don't have to feel guilty about that. It doesn't take away from the value you put on other areas of your life."

I let that sink in.

"When I was working, all the changes I made really took place after I clarified my values; what I felt were most important to me."

I nodded.

"So, with me," Jim continued, "I value Vanessa and my kids, and time with them is number one. I value my and our health, and having a sense of wellness. I value our social ties. I also value leadership. I've always loved being a leader. I worked into a position of leadership at work. Now, through being a volunteer, I get to teach and coach, and that's important to me. So, Alex, what's important to you? What do you value?"

Right away, I answered, "I value Joanie and David, so I guess my family relationships as well as those with my friends. That's my number one. I value being able to be active. I didn't realize how much I missed sports and activity, and all the camaraderie that goes with it."

I paused. "And I do value work. I'm good at it and I enjoy helping people and making sure my clients are successful."

"Then don't apologize for that," Jim counseled. "If you clarify your values, it will help you balance things, set your limits, and work toward your vision of what you want your life to be."

"Yeah, that makes sense," I said, half to myself. I paused. "Look, I'm not going to lie. I like nice stuff, too."

Jim nodded.

"One of my best friends is very unapologetic about his love of cars," Jim said. "It's one of the things that motivates him to work hard. He's got a really full life, and his Porsche and Jaguar are a part of it." Jim grinned.

"My brother can live out of a backpack," I told Jim. "He's all about new experiences."

"Yes, Vanessa and I are leaning more that way, too, these days," Jim said.

Jim added one last thing.

"This sounds kind of morbid, but a counselor told me once to imagine what I would want my eulogy to be. How would you want to be remembered? He was a great dad? Husband? He was a volunteer? He was the life of the party? He was a leader? It will help you focus on what you want out of life, your vision, and what's important to you."

That conversation was a huge lightbulb for me.

And the lunch was restorative.

I had a great afternoon - proactive and positive.

I did some research. Then, later that week, I walked into my boss's office and presented him with a list of some areas where we could be a healthier work environment, and be more efficient to boot. Some of them involved things I had started doing when I met Jim, then abandoned: active meetings, etc.

Honestly, in the back of my mind, I had a fear of being let go, but I knew I would land on my feet.

My boss looked skeptical at first, but after seeing all the research on how balance and wellness help keep people happy (and efficient) and, in turn, companies successful, he loved it. He also liked the idea of being seen as progressive.

Within a few days, we had changes in place. We started making water available and encouraged in the office. There was always a cooler of plain water, as well as cucumber and lemon slices, if anyone wanted some flavor. It cut down on the soft drinks and I started hearing lots of positive comments.

We fixed up our lunch room, and it became an unwritten rule that you didn't eat at your desk while working anymore. More than a few people commented that they felt better.

We ordered in a couple of adjustable stand-up desks (so people could stand or sit at them), on a trial basis, and they were a hit!

They were small changes, but they were making a big difference.

CHAPTER 43

Speaking of changes, Joanie, David and I had a big family meeting.

There was going to be a big change in our house: an addition to our family.

No, it was not the baby that my mother thought we should have. (Although that could still be a possibility.)

This involved a little girl by the name of Sunshine. She was blond and furry and sweet. She was an eight-week old retriever mix, who we fell in love with at the shelter.

We had started to talk about getting a dog over the summer, as we started to balance our lives.

One thing Joanie had been firm on, was that we couldn't have a dog if we didn't have time to properly care for him or spend time with her. That wouldn't be fair to the dog, and it would have added more stress to our household.

David, for a five year old, had some pretty convincing arguments though. And, the more we thought about what kind of lifestyle we wanted, the more a little canine family member seemed to fit.

Joanie and I, not wanting to get David's hopes up, had gone to look at the puppy, while one of our neighbors, a kind, outgoing teenager named Kylie, hung out with David.

(That was another change we had welcomed: a wonderful babysitter, so that Joanie and I could have date nights here and there. David loved Kylie, so it was win-win.)

Once we met the puppy, we knew she would be a good fit for us. She was energetic and affectionate.

So when we sat down to have our family meeting with David, and told him that we were going to have a new family member, he looked unimpressed at first.

When we described her and explained that she needed a family who would love her and take of her, he was as excited as I've ever seen him.

When we brought her home, he named her Sunshine right away.

"Isn't that going to be your wife's name when you grow up?" I asked, thinking back to our game.

"I don't need a wife when I have a puppy," he exclaimed, and we laughed.

We invited a couple of neighbors to meet Sunny. Kim and Ty's kids were all over her.

"Thanks man," Ty said, half-joking. "Now guess who's going to want a dog?"

David was so nurturing and protective of Sunny.

We were going to rescue her, as he told Jim and Vanessa, and, as David astutely put it, she was going to rescue us. From boredom, according to him.

I thought it might be a little more far reaching than that, although I didn't feel like I needed to be saved so much anymore. I did have someone to thank for starting the process. But I was finally saving myself.

CHAPTER 44

A couple of weeks later, David started school.

We walked him to school with Sunny. And we weren't offended when he gave her a bigger hug than us.

It was bittersweet. David looked so cute with his little backpack - so young, but like a little man at the same time.

He gave us both a final kiss and a wave, and he was off, into his classroom.

Joanie and I went out for a snack (with Sunny in tow) after dropping David off. We sat outside at a local café, meeting up with a few other parents who didn't know whether to be happy or sad about the first day of school.

We were really in the moment.

"Someday he'll be going off to college," I told Joanie. "And we'll wish we were back to this day, when he's just five years old. Let's enjoy it."

We did enjoy it. We had a happy kid. As we chatted with a few other parents, we realized we were about to be part of a nice community at his school.

David's first day of school brought back memories of my first day at school. I felt like such a big guy. My little brother cried. Emily and I were always close, but Richard was my little sidekick. Later, I was so proud to show him around when he started grade primary.

I called my brother that afternoon.

Richard was in Venezuela. After the initial surprise of hearing from me (I think I took him out of a meeting), it was like we were kids again. He couldn't believe David had started school. Rich told me about the project he was working on, and I told him how proud I was of him. With promises to re-connect (which we would keep), and with a gruff but sincere 'I love you' each way, we hung up.

That evening, we had a special dinner, and frozen yogurt sundaes, while David told us all about his "awesome day" at school.

That fall, we harvested a bunch of veggies from our garden, and settled into a routine with more balance.

David played basketball, and I loved helping coach.

Everyone in my office embraced the new focus on employee wellness we incorporated. A favorite was the stability balls that we got to sit on during meetings.

The only one who was hesitant to use them was Bryan, and that was after a little mishap. (Let me just say, you shouldn't try to see how high you can bounce on them!)

Bryan came on board afterward though. A little after he was diagnosed with an ulcer.

Efficiency at our office went up, and absenteeism went down. Work became a positive again.

Speaking of work, one day, a Monday, Will popped into my office, just to say hi. He was on one of his 'movement breaks' to clear his head.

"Hey, I think we're going to walk down to the ferry terminal tomorrow for lunch. There's a new sushi place. Want to join us?"

"Ah, love to," I replied, "but I usually meet Jim for lunch on Tuesdays. You should meet him sometime."

"Jim?"

"Remember? My neighbor that I told you about. Jim Chipman."

"That's funny," Will commented. "I did a profile in business school on James Chipman. But he worked in New York for a lot of his career."

"So did Jim," I said.

Will's eyes widened. "As a consultant?"

"Yeah," I nodded.

"James Chipman?" he repeated. "Also known as JC Chipman?!"

"Yeah," I confirmed. "You know. He lives across the street from me."

"James Chipman, the former CEO of KoMF Consulting?!" Will shot back. "*That's* Jim?"

"Uh," I started.

Will rushed to my desk.

"Look him up. Search 'James Chipman Business'!"

I woke up my laptop and entered Jim's name.

Holy crap.

Jim had successfully led a huge, and I mean mammoth global business management consulting company, working his way up to CEO. Then he left that and brought another one back from near ruin. The last one he led, KoMF, stood for 'Keep on Moving Forward'. Clever.

As I scrolled down, we saw articles and business magazine covers. He looked a little different back then. Maybe it was the suit and the slicked back hair. He looked kind of badass!

"That's Jim?" Will nearly screeched. "He's a legend, a total rock star!"

I was a little blown away.

"Wow, I had no idea. I didn't even know his last name until a while ago," I told Will. "Want to join us for lunch sometime?" I asked, grinning.

Will gave me his 'are you insane' look. "Uh, yeah."

"Okay, you'll really like him," I called after Will, as he got back to work.

CHAPTER 45

Fall drifted into winter.

I had a bit of travel with work. On one of the trips, to Boston, Joanie and David joined me, and we made a weekend out of it. (Sunshine got spoiled at Kim and Ty's place.)

I did invite Will to lunch with Jim and I, and, after he got over being a little star struck, we all had a great time.

I asked Jim later why he didn't tell me about being such a mover and shaker. (From what I read, he had made millions.)

His answer was simple:

"That's not what I value now, Alex."

I nodded, and I got it.

"The money makes us comfortable, and I was able to help our kids, but getting awards, or seeing my face on a magazine or buying expensive things are not what make me happy."

"That's really cool, Jim," I told him.

"But between you and I, I'm surprising Vanessa with a bike trip in Italy," he whispered excitedly. "That's what she and I want. Experiences that are meaningful."

"Mum's the word." I smiled.

Joanie and I made a conscious decision to focus on family and friends at Christmastime, and not so much 'stuff'. David was most excited about the bicycles we all got, and the 'indestructible' ball for Sunny.

We also set limits, guarding our own time. We went for walks with Sunny, and hot chocolate, played games, baked cookies, and spent lots of time with people we love. It was David's happiest Christmas, and ours too.

And then winter melted into spring.

Will and Ashley had a healthy, beautiful baby girl. Everyone at the office went in on one of those 'all-terrain' strollers, sort of like a baby jogger, so that they could be active with little Caroline.

We had them over a lot, and David loved her.

Sunshine grew like a weed, and David was so responsible with helping train her.

I wish I could say that, for us, everything went smoothly from then on, but of course there were challenges here and there.

That's life.

We set our priorities for balancing work with family life, eating well, being active, and having meaningful experiences. I didn't freak out anymore when we had a setback. We just got back on track.

It was somewhere around a year from the night I first met Jim.

I thought of it as we walked at our weekly lunch. We were talking about basketball, and he was asking me how it was going.

"I want to thank you," I told him.

"For what?"

"For rescuing me," I joked. (Although I was pretty serious!)

He patted me on the shoulder.

"You saved yourself, Alex," he said. He paused, grinning. "I was just a good coach."

I grinned back. I was really grateful for Jim's friendship, and his attitude and wisdom.

So grateful, in fact, that I swore to myself that I'd pass it on.

So. Here you go…

ARE YOU READY?
A GUIDE

Alex's story isn't far off from what happens to most of us, at some point in our lives.

We have the best intentions to 'live a great (and grateful) life'.

Media, commercials, books, and self-help gurus tell us we should have it all, and hold it together! Meanwhile, we're plugged in and 'on' 24/7.

We're driven to succeed. Yet, amid all the pressure to have the perfect life, who doesn't feel overwhelmed, at least once in a while?

It happens to the best of us.

It's not that difficult, or complicated, to live a fuller, happier life – on your terms.

Check out our chapter-by-chapter guide, and ask yourself:

Did you notice?

IN CHAPTER 1: HOPELESSNESS

Did you notice the sense of despair Alex felt?

He felt hopeless. When an individual loses his or her sense of control, it can result in a form of grief. That can prevent them from being objective and rational and can result in hopelessness. You can end up feeling stuck and not able to change. It's like a record skipping on a turntable.

Starting point: If you feel hopeless, it's important to get out of your head and understand that these are just stories and not reality. Make the decision to doubt your hopelessness. Simply entertain the notion that you could be wrong. Most who feel this kind of despair are overgeneralizing from a few experiences.

Quick tip: Make a list of past successes in the domain you feel hopeless in. Focus on past achievements to pull you through tough times.

CHAPTER 2: COPING SKILLS: ALCOHOL

Did you notice that Alex uses alcohol as a coping mechanism?

Alcohol can become a negative coping skill for stress.

Starting point: Cravings and urges are time-limited; that is, they usually last only a few minutes and at most a few hours. If you always have a drink at the end of the day, plan something else, like a walk with a friend or your partner.

Quick tip: Stock your house with drinks other than alcohol, like Perrier or other sparkling water, tonic water (great with lime), iced teas, herbal teas, etc. so you don't automatically turn to alcohol.

CHAPTER 3: MY ENVIRONMENT CONTROLS ME

Did you notice that Alex felt like he had lost control of his life?

People who operate from an external locus of control perceive the environment is controlling their choices.

Starting point: When you feel trapped, write down a list of all possible courses of action. Tap into your creativity.

Quick tip: It's helpful to remember that, while you can't control everything in your day, you <u>can</u> control how you respond to a situation or problem.

Quick tip: It's easy (and common) to feel like you're not even in control of your own schedule. Write it down. Spread out a calendar of your week, with each day broken into hours. Mark in the times that you have to be at work, or other 'must do's (like sleep). How much time is left each day? Will you use it for leisure? Time to be active or exercise? Take control of it.

CHAPTER 4: FAMILY UNITY

Did you notice how negative Alex was about his parents' visit, effectively changing his weekend plans?

Starting point: Have compassion for those around you. Set limits but remember they love you. Don't be afraid to have open conversations and set expectations. Know what you need out of the relationship and what they need.

Quick tip: Be a good communicator. Alex could sit down with his parents and wife, when his parents arrive, and talk. Don't be afraid to have an open and honest disucssion, whether it's about your relationship, schedule, or limits. Make a pact to start every visit with a 15 minute check in.

CHAPTER 5: ACCEPTANCE

Did you notice Alex's negative attitude and outlook during his parents' visit?

Starting point: Whether it's a situation you can't control, a personality trait that is hard to change, or an emotion that overwhelms, accepting it can allow you to move forward.

Quick tip: Accepting people allows for peace in your life.

CHAPTER 6: COPING SKILLS

Did you notice that Alex and his dad went straight for unhealthy fast food?

Emotional eating is the tendency to eat in times of stress, anxiety, anger, or sadness.

You need to find an alternative to these states.

Starting point: If you're down, have someone on speed dial to call and talk it out. If you're feeling anxious, commit to go for a walk or run prior to your sugar staple. Notice how many times you don't crave it anymore.

Quick tip: Next time you find yourself hungry in a food court, look around. What are the healthy alternatives to your usual fast food?

Did you notice how upset Alex's dad got over a scratch on the car?

It's easy to let even little things bother you, particularly when you're not feeling great. Remind yourself to look at the big picture.

Starting point: Do a quick perspective assessment: Is this going to bother me tomorrow? Next week? Next month? If not, it won't seem like such a big deal.

Quick tip: Dwelling on stuff takes up space in your brain, rent-free. If it's a problem you can fix or move forward on, great. If not, put it away, at least for a while.

Did you notice how Alex never gets a good night sleep anymore?

Starting point: Set a wind down schedule for yourself, and follow it when you can. Have a book or magazine at bedtime, that's just interesting enough (but doesn't keep you awake)!

Quick tip: Keep any electronics away from your bedroom and nighttime routine. When you can, turn them off and put them away. Allow yourself to unplug.

CHAPTER 7: STRESS NEVER LEAVES

Did you notice that Alex had fun at the neighborhood barbeque, even though he initially saw it as just another commitment?

Starting point: Remember that a healthy, productive person has meaningful relationships in their life. This is not just with family, but also socially. Having someone who cares about you and you can count on as a support will help in troubling times and help keep the good time rolling.

Quick tip: Compartmentalize your time. When you're at work, by all means, focus on work. When you're at a social event or having some downtime, don't let thoughts about work creep in. Be in the moment.

CHAPTER 8: PLANNING

Did you notice how Alex connected with his wife and son over supper?

Planned meals and planned time with those close to you will help you stay healthy.

Starting point: Planning your meals at the start of the week, and taking time out to enjoy them – at least a few times a week - will help you move forward with your health.

Quick tip: Preparing the meal is another time to connect. Give everyone a job, and enjoy being together while you get everything ready.

CHAPTER 9: STRESS EFFECT

Did you notice that Alex's friend, Will, talked about how stressful it was for his wife to get pregnant?

Starting point: Not being able to conceive can be stressful. Give yourself the best chance by stress reduction techniques like meditation, as stress elevates hormones counterproductive to encouraging pregnancy.

Quick tip: Try going to yoga together. Learn to meditate together. Try not to sweat the small stuff, because most of life is the small stuff.

CHAPTER 10: VOLUNTEER

Did you notice that Jim volunteers at the YMCA?

Volunteering provides physical and mental rewards. It reduces stress. When you reach out and focus on someone other than yourself, it interrupts usual tension-producing patterns.

Starting point: What are your interests? Coaching your kids' team? Fund-raising? Joining a service club? Nature and the environment?

Quick tip: Volunteering in an area you're interested in can put you in touch with others who share your values. (See Chapters 15 and 19!)

CHAPTER 11: COMMUNICATION

Did you notice how angry and frustrated Joan was in her conversation with Alex?

Two people can have different levels of skill when it comes to communication. Communication can improve and help grow your relationship.

Starting point: Consider getting a good book on communication skills. Try 'Just Listen'.

https://books.google.ca/books/about/Just_List en.html?id=YbFrqFfBQ0oC&source=kp_cover &redir_esc=y

Quick tip: Step one is good listening skills. When in a conversation, listen. Don't think about what you are going to say next. Be in the moment, and really try to understand what the other person is saying before you respond.

CHAPTER 12: NUTRITION ON THE GO

Did you notice the delicious and healthy food and drink Jim brought when he and Alex met for lunch?

Starting point: You can search out healthy fast food choices in your area on the web. Try apps like Yelp. Or ask around. (It's a great conversation starter!)

Or you can make something in your kitchen the night before.

Think of it as your own healthy fast food restaurant!

Quick tip: Get a bento box, and fill it with easy to grab food: almonds, berries, cheese, naan bread and dips… the list goes on! Have the easy stuff on hand at home, so you can grab it, even as a 'just in case' backup.

CHAPTER 13: NORMALIZING FAILURE

Did you notice, in Jim's story, it was his son who initially pushed him to make a change? He had been unhappy and frustrated too, but kept going on the proverbial treadmill – just like Alex.

(And just like many of us!)

Starting point: Know that it's normal to fail. This is how we learn. See failure as an opportunity, rather than proof you are 'no good'.

Quick tip: Next time you have a setback or failure, don't waste time with regret. Ask yourself: What can I change for next time?

CHAPTER 14: MEDITATIVE WALKING

Did you notice that Jim and Alex walk in the park after lunch?

Meditative walking is a chance to get outside of your thoughts.

Starting point: Get out for a short walk, preferably in a quieter area. You can use the experience of walking as your focus, your anchor. It's the opportunity to notice the wind, sun, rain, and the sounds of nature. It's easier to be in tune to your body while moving rather than sitting meditation.

Quick tip: Start by feeling the soles of your shoes hit the ground. Notice the sound and the feel. Listen to the wind or feel the warmth of the sunshine on your face.

CHAPTER 15: SOCIAL PRESSURE

Did you notice that Bryan razzed Alex for not joining them for the usual unhealthy lunch?

Starting point: Look for the people at work who seem to have healthy habits. Get to know them.

Quick tip: When changing a behavior, try to find social circles that emulate the change, and that mimic your values. Or just order the healthy stuff anyway! Chances are, others will follow your lead.

CHAPTER 16: VISION

Did you notice that Alex talked with Joan about the positive changes he wanted to make?

Establishing your vision will provide a clear mental picture of what you want your total health and life to be in the future. This can be used as the foundation for the motivation to continue on your journey to your future self.

Starting point: Write your own eulogy. It sounds morbid, but it will give you tremendous power over your life. Who do you want to be? What do you want to be known for?

Quick tip: With every decision or challenge, remind yourself of what your vision is. It will give you clarity, and hopefully, reduce anxiety.

CHAPTER 17: FIRST STAGE OF CHANGE

Did you notice that Alex and Joan made a list of their priorities?

When a person moves out of feeling hopeless, they become motivated to learn and do. This is the first step in moving toward a positive lifestyle.

Starting point: At this stage, often you are open to learn and develop skills needed for positive health. We can all struggle or even slip back to hopelessness. However, the key outcome at this point of change is to keep focused on the hope of success. See what's possible.

Quick tip: Don't overwhelm yourself. Start with one or two of the priorities and make them stick before moving on.

CHAPTER 18: OPPORTUNITIES TO CONNECT

Did you notice that Alex enjoyed a pleasant breakfast with David and Joanie?

Starting point: We know that you can't always sit around having a leisurely breakfast! But, when you can, take the time – even if it's an extra five or fifteen minutes to sit down, eat mindfully (as opposed to gobbling something fast while on the run) and connect with your partner, your kid, or your friends. It will enhance your life - and theirs.

Quick tip: Pick a time that works best for you. For some it may be breakfast or lunch, for others, evening will be better. Pick which one makes you feel the least rushed.

CHAPTER 19: PEER PRESSURE ROUND 2

Did you notice that Alex is re-thinking who he wants to surround himself with and how he wants to spend his time?

Starting point: To deal with the pressure, be clear on what values are important to you; and choose your friends wisely. Seek out people at work who seem to have active, healthy habits.

Quick tip: Volunteering (coaching, environmental groups, etc.) or joining a club or sport group are just a couple of ways to surround yourself with people who have common values with you.

CHAPTER 20 – BRIGHT OR STORMY WEATHER

Did you notice that Alex asked Jim if they should change lunch because of potential bad weather?

Starting point: Being prepared for alternatives when trying to change your physical activity behavior is important. We suggest developing a set of regular activities that are always available regardless of weather. (indoor cycling, aerobics, swimming, mall walking, dancing…)

Quick tip: The Norwegians say that there's no bad weather - only bad clothing. Get yourself some decent gear for rain, snow, or whatever weather you get to deal with!

CHAPTER 21: RELATIONSHIP PLANNING

Did you notice that Alex and Joanie are practical and realistic about what they can change?

Starting point: Buying a calendar and noting important activities and dates is a great step forward.

Quick tip: Make a pact with your partner that you'll talk, take twenty minutes to connect in the evening, text, or whatever works to make your relationship a priority, even if your week is crazy.

CHAPTER 22 – NUTRITION: THE HEALTHY CHOICE

Did you notice that Alex made a healthy choice for his lunch with Jim?

Sometimes you have to eat out, and sometimes you want to eat out!

That's okay.

Starting point: There are so many fantastic options these days for take-out, and restaurants in general. (Get to know someone like Mimi!)

Quick tip: If you 'fall off the wagon' and make some unhealthy choices, don't beat yourself up about it. Look forward and make better choices next time!

(AND, ONE MORE TIME!)
CHAPTER 22: MENTOR

Did you notice that Jim has become a true mentor to Alex?

Who can be your mentor? A Yoda to your Luke Skywalker.

What separates a mentor from others in your life is a long term commitment and a keen investment in your future.

Starting point: Who do you admire at work? School? In your community? Invite them for coffee. Chances are, they'll take it as a compliment.

Quick tip: You can have a few mentors. Perhaps you have a favorite college professor, your boss from your first job, or someone at work.

CHAPTER 23:
SOCIAL CIRCLES

Did you notice that even David is becoming aware of being around people who make "bad choices"?

Fitting in feels good, even at the expense of your otherwise good sense. **Starting point:** Avoidance in the beginning may be the right advice. If you don't like who you are or what you do around certain people, try to bypass those social situations.

Quick tip: Be okay to bow out of plans that don't feel right to you.

CHAPTER 24: THE VOICE IN MY HEAD

Did you notice that Alex felt like Bryan thought he was being slack?

It is a natural human condition to think the worst.

Starting point: You need to break the cycle of consistently evaluating yourself through your thoughts. Next time you catch yourself thinking the worst, stop and give yourself an optimistic or positive thought to chew on.

Quick tip: Read up on cognitive diffusion. Cognitive diffusion consists of encouraging yourself to detect your thoughts, and to see them as hypotheses rather than objective facts about the world.

CHAPTER 25: THE WEEKEND IS THE WEEKEND

Did you notice how revitalized Alex and his family were once they decided to relax and enjoy their weekend?

Starting point: What do you do to relax and have fun on the weekend? Plan something enjoyable to keep your mind away from work.

Quick tip: If you have a family, give everyone a weekend to decide an activity. Maybe you choose bowling, your partner chooses a hike, your daughter wants to go swimming, etc.

If you have a group of friends, you can do the same thing. (It's also a great way to try a new activity.)

Quick tip: Have a spot to put your phone away, or turn it on mute when you don't need it. That one simple act will eliminate distractions, and allow you to focus on your weekend. (Works great for evenings too!)

CHAPTER 26: WORKOUT BUDDY

Did you notice that Alex said yes to going to the fitness center with Jim?

Having a workout buddy has been shown to increase adherence.

Starting point: Take advantage of someone else's drive to get your motivation up.

Quick tip: Don't know anyone who works out at your interest/level? Try putting it out there on social media. Ask who knows great places to work out in your area, near work, etc. Are there any new gyms, spin and fitness studios, or classes your friends have tried? Chances are, you'll get lots of positive feedback.

Quick tip: Look into clubs. What's your interest? Between running, cycling, and hiking clubs, racquet and other sport clubs... and social activity groups for adults, there are a lot of options.

CHAPTER 27: THE MANY FORMS OF MEDITATION

Did you notice how proud David was of their garden?

We discussed walking meditation but it can come in other forms.

Some see gardening as a form of meditation. The simple acts of planting, weeding, having your hands in the soil, etc. make you focus on your environment – one that you're creating.

Starting point: Meditation doesn't have to mean sitting in a garden, or on a mat, holding your index fingers to your thumbs. (If that's your style, that's great too.) The goal is to be in the moment. Start by taking five slow, deep breaths. Tune out everything else. Focus on the air going in through your nose, and out through your mouth.

Quick tip: You can meditate anywhere. Close your door at your office, and take a few minutes to zone out everything else, and just breathe.

(See Chapter 35.)

CHAPTER 28: SITTING

Did you notice that Alex, Joanie, and their friends got up and walked around the garden, etc. at dinner?

Prolonged sitting is the new smoking.

Starting point: Think of how you can get more movement in your life, whether it's at home or at work.

Is it walking meetings, getting out of the car to get your coffee, or biking to work?

Quick tip: Remember this line, next time you need to meet with someone or come up with an idea: "I think better when I walk."

(And by the way, most of us do think better when we move!)

CHAPTER 29: GOOD SOCIAL CIRCLES

Did you notice that Alex and Joanie are starting to re-connect with people who share the same values as them?

Starting point: Whatever behavior you're thinking of changing, think of a group that would be supportive, and join in.

Quick tip: Remember, people are happy to be invited, whether it's an outing, or a meal. It doesn't have to take a lot of effort. Best invention ever: the potluck. It's easy, everyone is happy to contribute, and you'll probably end up with some great new food ideas!

CHAPTER 30: GET HELP

Did you notice that Jim talked about meeting with a personal trainer to help him get fit and active?

Starting point: Whether it's a nutritionist, psychologist, or personal trainer, get professional help.

Quick tip: Everyone loves to talk about how great their trainer is (we hope!) or their physical therapist, etc. Ask around.

Quick tip: If you don't have a primary care physician, get one. In a lot of cases, that's your 'square 1' to getting/staying healthy.

CHAPTER 31: HAVE FUN

Did you notice that Alex started playing basketball again, a sport that he loved in school?

Starting point: Do some reminiscing and look back to where you were committed. What activity motivated you?

Quick tip: Or try something new! You probably know people who have tried sports or activities like skiing, golf, tennis, running or hiking as adults, and fell in love with them. The sky's the limit!

CHAPTER 32: VOLUNTEERING: PART 2

Did you notice that Alex is excited about helping coach basketball?

Starting point: If you can tie your volunteering to your family, or to an activity you already love, that's terrific.

Coaching a child's sport team is a super example (as long as it's a positive experience for you AND your child).

Quick tip: Start by figuring out what is realistic for you to commit to and what you are passionate about.

For some it might be walking dogs at the SPCA one night a week, for others coaching a team 4 nights a week. Make sure you can fully commit without feeling stressed or overcommitted.

CHAPTER 33: CAREER

Did you notice, while playing The Game of Life, Joanie starts to talk about what kind of work she'd like to do?

Starting point: Do you know what your values are? Don't be on the countdown to retirement. Whether it's making a move within your profession or company, or doing something completely different, think about what drives you. Start creating a plan today to move towards a fulfilling career.

Quick tip: Go to a career counselor. There are also plenty of websites where you can do mini-assessments and find out what may peak your interest.

CHAPTER 34: FAMILY

Did you notice how good it feels for Alex and his sister (and their families) to re-connect?

Starting point: Positive family relationships are 25 percent of resilience. Pick up the phone and check in on a family member.

Quick tip: You can connect with your family on your terms. If you love your family, but hate the annual get together, suggest or plan something else.

CHAPTER 35: MINDFULNESS

Did you notice how Alex is able to stop and be mindful of his surroundings?

Starting point: Mindfulness is simply focusing on what you're doing now - breathing, watching the birds in the park, noticing the sun's warmth on your face – without being barraged by other thoughts. It's a way to increase living in the present, which relieves anxiety and depression. (There's a reason the old saying, 'Stop and smell the roses' became a cliché.)

Quick tip: Remember there is neither a right nor wrong way to be mindful. Leave the judgement and evaluation on the shelf and start your practice today.

CHAPTER 36: THE WINDY ROAD

Did you notice how defeated Alex feels when things tighten up at work?

Sometimes, as they say, life gets in the way. If you get bumped off the road to feeling better, don't feel beat yourself up. Just step back on.

Maintain your hope, determination and self confidence in trying times. The key is to know your vision and values.

Starting point: When you fall, as you're getting up, read your vision statement and remember who you are and what is important to you.

Quick tip: When you're working toward a goal, enjoy the process. See failures as comforting, because you're learning from them. See lapses or setbacks as building blocks.

Things got crazy at work and home, and you fell off that perfect exercise schedule? Every setback makes you a little wiser. What strategies will you use next time?

CHAPTER 37: TAKE A DEEP BREATH

Did you notice that Alex stopped to take a deep breath?

Starting point: An age-old tradition: Stop as many times as you need to in a day, and take 5 big belly deep breaths and notice the difference.

Start by getting into a comfortable position, whether lying or sitting. Close your eyes if you like and start by relaxing your shoulders. If thoughts come into your head, be okay with that. Let them drift away like a leaf in the wind. Slowly inhale, feeling the air move along the path of your nostrils and into your lungs. Keep it slow and intentional. Hold it for a second and slowly exhale out your mouth feeling in move across your lips. Start to scan your body while doing this, looking for tight muscles.

Quick tip: Put it in your schedule and do not book over it. Give yourself 5 minutes everyday. Put in a time that works for you.

CHAPTER 38: THE NEW AGE OF WORK

Did you notice how Jessica called the work environment "toxic"?

…And the company lost a talented employee because her need for flexibility was seen as a negative.

Many companies are learning the value of allowing employees to work at home, have flexible hours and a more relaxed work environment.

Starting point: To suggest flexible hours (or other morale boosting changes), if you have an idea, gather the positives and talk to your boss today.

Quick tip: If you are leader, can you let your employees choose their time to work, or even some flexibility? Have a meeting specifically to discuss this. Some people are happier and more efficient early in the day; others work better from 6 to 8 p.m. at night, and also enjoy it more.

When your team is positive and productive, that's a win for everyone.

CHAPTER 39: BOUNCE BACK

Did you notice that Alex has a major set-back?

The ability to bounce back, from big or little failures, is a huge tool in your personal toolbox.

Starting point: When a set-back hits, think: *What can I learn from this? How can I maneuver around this kind of thing next time?*.

Become a strategic analyst.

Quick tip: Remember this: If your favorite team quit every time they lost, there would be one team left in the league. Failure is normal. Like your favorite high-level athlete, learn from it and move on.

CHAPTER 40: IT'S NOT WORK-LIFE BALANCE. IT'S LIFE.

Did you notice that Alex falls back into old habits at work?

Starting point: If you love your work, and you want it to be a big slice, don't feel guilty. It's fantastic to be passionate about what you do!

If you don't love your work, try to get a smaller slice, or change the pie! It doesn't mean you have to walk in and quit tomorrow, but you can start to look at professional development options in your field, or polish your resume and look around.

Quick tip: Do a self-performance review every three months: Am I enjoying my life? Am I getting what I want out of my career?

Also have a sit down with your family and do a check-in to make sure everyone's needs are getting met.

CHAPTER 41: OPTIMISM AND RESILIENCE

Did you notice that Jim talks about the importance of bouncing back, a theme that has come up more than once?

Starting point: The biggest part of being resilient is maintaining optimism.

We all have catastrophic thinking, where we imagine the worst case scenario. Be okay with it, and allow yourself to do it briefly, so you can think of solutions. But don't dwell on it. Then let yourself think of the opposite scenario: What if this all works out in my favor? What does the positive look like?

Quick tip: Try writing it. Keep a journal.

CHAPTER 42: IF YOU WANT CHANGE…

Did you notice that Alex did some research on a better work environment, and then went to his boss with it?

Starting point: If you don't ask or communicate, how can you expect change? Talk to your coworkers and your boss.

Ask to start a wellness action team at your place of employment.

From here, search out a good assessment tool. (If you're looking for examples, Howatt HR has an excellent assessment tool for quality of work life, or QWL.)

You can hone in on the needs of your group. After this, you can set out an action plan to start to improve the group's total health.

Quick tip: Creating a healthy, active workplace empowers everyone, and leads to a positive work environment. Even small changes (like the water or lunchroom) can lead to big results. People feel supported, and you end up with a dynamic workforce.

Watch how people buy into it.

CHAPTER 43: WHO LET THE DOGS OUT?

Did you notice that Joanie was adamant that they would only get a dog if they had time and energy for one?

Dogs bring a lot of joy to a house, as do pets in general.

Adopting a dog or cat is a commitment for the life of your new 'fur kid'. Make sure you have the time and the resources (people to help if you travel, etc.)

Starting point: Write down the pros and cons of having a pet and make an informed decision. Ask lots of questions. (People love to talk about their pets.) If you want a dog, do some research on which breed is best. If you have a family, make sure everyone's on board (and ready to do leash duty)!

Quick tip: If you're not sure you're ready for a pet at this point in your life, volunteer to take care of a friend's dog while they're away, or lend a hand at your local SPCA.

CHAPTER 44 AND 45: WHAT DO YOU VALUE?

Did you notice that Alex came back to what he values?

By the end of the story, we know that he values his family. He values his health and wellness. He values his friends. And yes, he values his career.

Getting to know someone outside his or her career can be a profound experience. Asking someone: *What do you value? What are you grateful for?* or *Who do you admire?* rather than *What do you do for a living?* opens up a whole new relationship and perspective.

Alex learned this in the end.

Would their relationship have been the same if Alex knew Jim was a guru in the profession? Would he have been as open?

Value-based living is what we believe helps us live a more meaningful life. It makes life decisions easier and also keeps us grounded.

Do you know what you value?

Are your decisions in line with your values?

Whether this book is a game changer for you, or it gave you a couple of lightbulb moments, we hope you can take a piece of Alex's story and use it in yours. Here's to your future.

FOR MORE INSIGHTS AND TIPS, CHECK OUT:

www.vendurawellness.com
www.incitewellness.ca
And on Twitter….
@VenduraWellness

Other Resources
HR solutions:
www.howatthr.com

Leadership training:
www.visioncoachinginc.com
www.bluteaudevenney.com

Corporate health assessments:
http://www.morneaushepell.com/ca-en/total-health-index

Motivational speaking:
www.markdejonge.com
http://www.ipromiseperformance.com/speaking/

ACKNOWLEDGEMENTS
AND THANKS

From Darren:
Thanks to Phil Campagna for helping me get into school, and being a mentor like no other. Amir Nevo for his outstanding insight, suggestions and encouragement. Janice MacInnis who has been a colleague for nearly 20 years and is always providing a helping hand. To Keith Abriel, Greg Caines, and Bill Howatt, who are leaders in their fields, many thanks for your guidance. Mark de Jonge, an amazing role model, thanks for your feedback. Jesse Adams my partner in crime, Kent, Terry, Coach McGarrigle, my brother Dannie, my sister Dana, and my parents for always being there. All the sports coaches I learned from as an athlete. And of course, Julia, who has supported me in everything I try, and loves me unconditionally.

From Sue:
Thanks to those who read the book in its various stages, and gave us such amazing guidance, especially Amir Nevo. I'm not sure how many times we said, "Let's run it by Amir," but it was

more than a few.

Sven Grabke, thank you for your (as usual) sage advice.

Tom Stender, for your keen eye, thanks buddy, and happy sailing.

Thanks to Mom, for always telling me I could do anything, and Dave and Randy, for always having my back.

My dad was a successful small town businessman, and an even better parent. He taught my brothers and me the value of connecting, and a good story. Thanks, Dad. I miss you.

Mark, Tom and Carolina, and Skyler, who motivate me everyday. Love you guys!

ABOUT THE AUTHORS

Darren Steeves is passionate about improving the total health of our community. Darren is a Certified Exercise Physiologist with a Masters degree in kinesiology and a Bachelors degree in education. He has worked in the health and performance field for over 20 years. He is a co-owner of *Vendura Wellness*, a health consulting company and sole owner of Steeves Training Systems providing one on one coaching to executive coaches.

Darren is an adjunct professor in the School of Health and Human Performance at Dalhousie University, conducting research in the areas of resilience, and performance measures in high performance sport. He has consulted within corporations, with top-level executives, Olympic Medalists and World Champion athletes, and has attended the Olympic games as a sport scientist with Team Canada. Darren was also one of the original authors of Behavioural Engineering, the theory behind an innovative IT solution, called *Incite*, for use in corporations with employees.

Darren lives in Halifax, Nova Scotia with his wife, Julia and dog Rudy and enjoys their walks, talks (and barks) at the park on the weekends.

Sue Comeau has been interested in attainable wellness and fitness since her days as a kinesiology student at Dalhousie University. Sue earned her Masters in exercise physiology from The University of North Carolina at Chapel Hill. She's a Certified Exercise Physiologist with the Canadian Society for Exercise Physiology.

She has taught wellness, exercise prescription, and program design in Dalhousie University's School of Health and Human Performance, as a lecturer.

After years of writing on health and fitness, and writing fiction, Sue combined the two. She is the author of *The F.I.T. Files*, which uses narrative to promote fitness and healthy living for kids.

Sue lives in Halifax, Nova Scotia with her husband, two kids, and their Labrador retriever (kid #3).

Stop by and see **Sue at www.fitfiles.net**
Or on Twitter: @sue_comeau